THE RECLAIMED WOMAN

THE

LOVE YOUR SHADOW

RECLAIMED

EMBODY YOUR FEMININE GIFTS

WOMAN

EXPERIENCE THE SPECIFIC PLEASURE OF WHO YOU ARE

KELLY BROGAN, MD

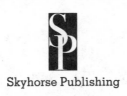

Skyhorse Publishing

Skyhorse Publishing books may be purchased in bulk at special discounts for sales promotion, corporate gifts, fund-raising, or educational purposes. Special editions can also be created to specifications. For details, contact the Special Sales Department, Skyhorse Publishing, 307 West 36th Street, 11th Floor, New York, NY 10018 or info@skyhorsepublishing.com.

Skyhorse® and Skyhorse Publishing® are registered trademarks of Skyhorse Publishing, Inc.®, a Delaware corporation.

Visit our website at www.skyhorsepublishing.com.

Please follow our publisher Tony Lyons on Instagram @tonylyonsisuncertain.

10 9 8 7 6 5 4 3 2 1

Library of Congress Cataloging-in-Publication Data is available on file.

Cover design by Skye High Interactive

Print ISBN: 978-1-5107-8070-5
Ebook ISBN: 978-1-5107-8071-2

Printed in the United States of America

To my parents, Ron & Marusca Brogan, for giving me this one wild life and affording me the perfect opportunities to choose to live it fully. And to my epic daughters, Sofia and Lucia Fink, who inspire every step of the path I walk home to myself.

Contents

Introduction

Words cannot express. . . .
I don't know how to describe . . .
I cannot even begin to explain. . . .

These are the messages I received from the women who attended my live event, Audacious Embodiment . . . and this is what happens when you come home to yourself as a woman:

   . . . you stop thinking
   . . . you stop explaining
   . . . you stop making a case for why you feel what you feel
And you simply FEEL.

The night after the event, I sat in the quiet of my home, leaned into my soft couch, and a tidal wave of feeling surfaced. Just like the other attendees, I felt disoriented and broken open . . .

I began to sob. Loud, ugly crying that I'd only ever experienced from pain and grief. Of course, I've shed tears of joy. I've held ecstasy in my body as streams ran down my face.

But this was different.

This was something I can only describe as love: eternal, universal embrace, delivered through my body.

I sobbed with the intensity of this energy moving through me like a geyser. This way of being with, truly feeling, and honoring embodied sensations is the central essence and power source of a Reclaimed Woman. It's how pleasure can be accessed in the here and now, inviting erotic life force to flow, so that life itself, knottiest challenges included, becomes an occasion for delight.

Here's what this luscious life looks like: You wake up without an alarm, pleased with the feeling of silk on your skin. You sense what your body wants in this moment, and you oblige, running your hands, slowly, up and down your belly. Throughout the rest of your day, you ask your body what she wants and are a custodian of her needs. You care for this body like a devoted lover: anointing, adorning, and honoring. When sensations and feelings arise, you know exactly how to attend to them, allowing them to transform into creative ideas and expressions. You make decisions with ease and confidence. You expect delight, synchronicity, and magic to effervesce from your life. You have tools and are *fully* equipped; you know when you're playing the age-old game of what I like to call "buying eggs from the hardware store," you wear the villain crown like a gorgeous evil queen, and you enter through the upset like a deep-sea explorer. You've got you. You're there for you. You love you. All of you. The anxiety, the depression, the agitation and vigilance melt. Your relationships are real. You fucking love being alive.

I'm going to be real with you; *I did not* live like this for most of my life. As a woman, I've been conditioned to self-betray and self-deny, just like you. But I've spent a long time on the magic carpet ride of reclamation, and I've learned about the sheer vibrancy that emerges when we open the permission field and create the conditions to fully enjoy the essence of the feminine. Let me take you back a decade, to 2014 . . .

My Reclaimed Woman Story (So Far)

I used to think I was confident.

Cool, comfortable, aloof, disaffected, I could slay a to-do list, or five, before breakfast. Like so many women of my generation, I was praised for getting good grades, for excelling, for problem-solving, productivity, and performance: all the masculine virtues. So, I developed what one of my absolute heroes, a genius of the polarity space, David Deida, calls a "masculine shell." But since a woman's masculine shell repels a masculine-essence man, I adorned myself with a feminine shell on top of my masculine shell. Hustling hard with perfect lipstick and a regular blowout (seriously, look at my old YouTubes). Over the years, my masculine shell hardened into rigidity, assuming a stiff shape with a tight belly, shoulders, and even a vagina clenched at rest. As the art of emotional alchemy was not modeled for me, I never really developed a relationship to my own emotions, which I generally regarded as problems to be fixed. The real me hid in the basement of my awareness as I applied proverbial staples, rubber bands, tape, and super glue to the mask of my persona. I became a masterful reactor, solution-finder, and a litigator-level self-defender. The vigilance I experienced became addictive, and rather than delighting in my body's desires, I'd spend my mornings scanning my lifescape for what was wrong.

This drive to fix every problem led me to clinical psychiatry, where it was promised that I could fix the problem of being human. Yet, despite sailing through M.I.T., Cornell, and N.Y.U., there were rumbles of rupture, sometimes called cognitive dissonance, that began to shake my insides when I opened my private practice. I remember sitting in my Madison Avenue office in Manhattan, across from a rather pregnant patient, rather pregnant myself. As I informed her of the relative safety of continuing her Zoloft prescription during her pregnancy, a voice inside me whispered: *I would never take that medication as a pregnant woman.* Well, that advice was inconvenient, since I had just completed my training as one of the first three hundred reproductive psychiatrists in the world, specializing in prescribing psychotropic medications to pregnant and breastfeeding women. *I'll just pretend that voice is the sound of a garbage truck outside and carry on.*

During this same year, I started researching birth interventions, reading tons of scientific literature about the known risks and unquantified concerns of hospitalized births, and ultimately decided that *I* wanted to have an intervention-free birth. Shocking, because I was certainly not any kind of Earth Mama. I was eating McDonalds for lunch, candy for dinner, and driving my system with roughly six cups of coffee a day. Based on my research, however, I discovered that less than 30 percent of obstetrical interventions are evidence-based.[1] *What?! How dare those OBs!* I defiantly switched to a midwife (more of a med-wife) and committed to a natural birth. In retrospect, I wish I had known even *one* home birthing woman to have expanded my activation of choice because until we know what is possible, we can only choose from what is known.

Ultimately, my first birth felt like a competitive *F You . . .* and *I'll show these OBs that I'm tough enough and don't need what they're peddling.* I set out on a marathon of *proving.* As I charged through seventeen hours of back labor, unmedicated, in a birth center, my allegiance to Mommy Medicine started to waver.

Fast forward, ten months postpartum, the rupture deepened, and my initiation journey fully ignited. With symptoms I could have easily written off as "new mom nuttiness," I felt like I was floating above myself most of the time. I forgot my ATM pin number, double booked patients, and waded through a fog that rolled in and out of my mind. During a routine physical, I was diagnosed with Hashimoto's Thyroiditis, a chronic, "incurable" disease that would "require" me to take medication for the rest of my life. I frantically searched for an exit door from the very system that I had been trained to support. A system that told me: *Sadly, you're sick. Be a responsible good girl and take your medication so you can get back to normal.*

I confronted a fork-in-the-road choice between taking Synthroid for the rest of my life or going out into the proverbial wilderness and seeing what would happen if I took the vision quest into the wild unknown (which, in the heroine's journey, appears after the threshold of a big *No* has been crossed). My Hashimoto's diagnosis initiated me to the adult reclamation of my health, my vitality, and ultimately my self-alignment.

You might imagine that I would have been shooting off fireworks of celebration when, through naturopath-recommended lifestyle change, I put my Hashimoto's into remission. Instead, I started launching grenades. My rage had been uncorked, my projections in full force, and I was going to take down this system that had betrayed me, lied to me, and worked me to the bone for crumbs. I was on the warpath, furious that I had never been taught that you could actually resolve the root cause of illness. That what you eat matters and so does every choice you make. That you actually *are* in control of your health, rather than some hapless victim at the mercy of bad genes, bad luck, and bad timing.

I took out a two-million-dollar life insurance policy and launched my activist career, published a grassroots *New York Times* bestseller with an exploding pharmaceutical pill on the cover, and dedicated myself to facilitating the liberation of women from the abusive allopathic system. My righteous bitch era was what I would now refer to as an adolescent stage of individuation. This stage is profoundly necessary, however, because it pushes you forward, beyond the habitual, the patterns, and the identity, into the fertile terrain of an expanded self. But it is *not* the destination.

Just when I settled into my new "awakened" identity as an anti-Pharma world-saver, I met my beloved mentor, Dr. Nicholas Gonzalez. At the time, I was crying myself to sleep at night about how totally bereft we all are and how wretched this world is, lamenting that I had brought children into this hellscape. Nick single-handedly reconnected my mission to my heart, to meaning, and to faith. His fierce conviction that the body does not make mistakes and his history-making outcomes in cancer and degenerative disease brought tears to my eyes, and when he suddenly passed, only a year into our journey together, another rupture ripped through the movie screen of my life. This time, an unmendable hole was torn in my activist identity. Brought to my knees with grief, I chose to honor him, and myself, by shifting my attention away from the angry, embittered fight, and toward the celebration of what's possible. I refined my

Vital Mind Reset health reclamation protocol, infusing it with his wisdom, and I set about igniting *Yes*'s in women all across the plane. I published my own history-making outcomes, conducted a randomized clinical trial of Vital Mind Reset to evidence these outcomes, and disrupted the dominant narrative around chronic illness, lifelong meds, and the identification with "sickness."[2]

Rupture: When I Lit My Reputation on Fire

You might think that this is where my reclamation story ends, but in many ways, health reclamation was just the beginning. Despite accumulating accolades, credentials, and evidence to *prove* that I was "right," I always kept my sights trained on the next dangling carrot, never to settle, never to rest, always imagining that I would finally feel okay when the next problem was solved. Obviously, my sense of worthiness required external evidence, and I clung to credibility-boosting data points like a life raft in the wild ocean, especially when my boat rocked. My clear opinions, my academic pedigree, my clinical expertise, my roles as wife, mother, daughter, sister, and activist were all rafts of virtue, and virtue-signaling, that I strapped onto my back.

Until life as I knew it ended, again.

The rupture that catalyzed my Reclaimed Woman journey began with the choice to leave my second marriage in 2021. There were parts of me that exploded over weeks of grief, anguish, and devastation. There were other parts of me that began to peek out from the cage I had locked them into, asking: *Is the coast clear?* Many of those softly questioning inner child parts demanded my attention.

One morning, after hours of moving in and out of a swirling abyss of grief, I felt a stirring to move my body. To dance. To express. It felt something like warm honey dripping down my belly. I felt an impulse to *record* myself, to be meta-witnessed by the all-seeing eye. An almost taunting, daring invitation to *expose* this dimension of myself, publicly, loudly, in creative celebration . . .

In a moment that was simultaneously so trivial and also life-defining, I chose to cut the cord to the biggest life raft I had at my disposal: my reputation.

From some perspectives, "reputation" is the highest value to the masculine. By willfully disidentifying with mine as my priority, I was ultimately accepting an opportunity to initiate my masculine through a kind of death-defying ritual, and thus to align more authentically with my feminine expression and desire. As I let the music move my hands over my body and swirl my hips, I wasn't consulting a spreadsheet of pros and cons; I was honoring a little "yes" inside. One that said: *Get out of this bed. Put on that song, the one with the BASS. Now move like you're making love to yourself . . .*

For another gal, posting a solo dance video might not have been anything more than a Saturday morning share. But for your lab-coat wearing, Ivy League–educated physician who was historically *very* careful not to show skin, curse, or share her erotic energy publicly, this social media ritual was the beginning of a new chapter. *Would I be stoned to death?* I jumped off the proverbial cliff. Without a parachute. In a bikini.

Within twenty seconds of clicking "post" on my video creation, energy rushed up my chest and neck. My stomach flipped. All of my inner self protectors were on red alert: *Just delete it. Nothing to see here. Are you actually crazy?!*

Another, righteous voice within me shouted: *You are doing this for other women too. It's important!*

Then there was another voice.

Softer. Gentler. One I hadn't heard in a while.

A little girl who simply said: *I love dancing, look at me!*

And so I did. Look at her. Finally.

I trained my gaze on my inner girl. From then on out, I decided to take care of her every impulse, creation, and request to express. I could also see more clearly than ever the parts of me that wanted to self-protect and self-preserve. I could appreciate their very valid and honorable intent, because it is forever their responsibility to make sure that I am never perceived as bad and wrong.

Over the ensuing months, I grew my capacity to hold these disparate parts, created space for them to express, and listened to their stories. I discovered that they had established a consensus around my sensuality and sexuality as energy to be "used" rather than embodied. I learned that I was living separately, almost self-objectified, from my erotic energy, and that this energy was distributed in discrete amounts, only when other protectors were led to believe that it was an "appropriate time" to allow for such a dispensation. When I leaned into the experience of my body as erotic by her very nature, I found great pleasure available to me, at any time, through dance. Like so many women before me, raw, open, and ready, I found myself with my soon-to-be calloused hand on a stainless-steel pole, in the back of a studio in Miami, with my angel of a girlfriend, Eyla. I fell for pole dancing fast and hard, literally and figuratively, for the months that ensued. I fell in love with my own energy moving through me, audaciously, sweetly, softly, strongly. And every time I would learn a dance routine, choose a costume, pick a song and edit it to a creative sound or poem, I felt like my five-year-old self, fingertips wet from a fresh painting.

One fateful day, I posted a video of myself in a pink bikini with leg warmers, playing into feminine slowness, moving around a pole as if I were swimming in honey. I had been so in my creative chamber of a cocoon that I didn't anticipate the degree to which my own residual shame would be mirrored back to me from my audience.

I have always been a provocateur, and I never experienced much inner disturbance when others disagreed with my intellectual, scientific, or clinical ideas. But this was *personal*.

Complete strangers posted comments like this:

"Totally not into this as something to broadcast to the world. I don't want to see you in your underwear. Some things are for privileged eyes only, a little discrimination needs to be brought to the table here."

"Am really put off by the pole dancing videos . . . it devalues what you are meant to stand for . . . do it on your own but not for your platform. Sorry I have unfollowed."

"NOTHING classy about flaunting it . . . It's about morals, modesty and values. Do these things still exist? This is something to do in the privacy of your own home and/or for your husband. If there's no line, then it will be crossed, and you may as well be pole dancing with half your arse hanging out to thousands of people watching online. Oh wait . . . "

And frankly, I felt truth in their collective outcry, "She's gone too far this time!"

Never a woman to delete or self-censor, I allowed the post to ferment like some kind of sour fruit (that I could only hope would mature into something palatable, at some point), and I walked into the terrifying cave of my inner turmoil.

Importantly, I *entered through the upset*, and I stayed with my body. I felt a round red spiky ball in the center of my chest that wanted me to defend myself with all sorts of high-minded and craftily-worded condemnations, with a touch of Jersey sass, about my commenters' sexual repression. The gooey blue blob traveling up my right side thought I could rally support from other sympathetic hearts by sharing the sad tale of those who turned against me. The black knife-like shape down by my lower left hip said: *You are an attention-seeking, deluded slut airing her midlife crisis on national television! Stop immediately.*

As soon as I honored all of these voices, I saw her once again. The tender child part within that they were all protecting, in their own way. I saw the little girl who just wants to play, to feel seen, understood, and celebrated. I wept with the innocence and sweetness of this part of me and the invisibility she has suffered with . . . invisible, chiefly, to me.

From this leap of faith, hurtling my reputation into the abyss, and the feeling of "I've made a mess too big to clean up," a fresh, new creative impulse was liberated in the direction of my highest expression. I spent an entire afternoon creating a video caricature of the woman who listens to what everyone else thinks she should do and be. After trying to stretch herself in a million directions, the ever-accommodating good girl ends up with duct tape across her mouth, head-to-toe clothing—*gotta have full coverage!*—a professional white lab coat, and a computer in front of her for good measure.

By the time I posted this tongue-in-cheek takedown of the new me, I had officially reclaimed aliveness in my body. Some essential aspect of my soul was given a perfect-sized place to rest. Behind the shame of "I've woman-ed wrong" was a longing to simply be in the lightness of my own ever-effervescing essence. And in that beingness, there's nothing to prove. There's no one to correct, and there's the delight of whatever the hell actually *is* happening. Truly. Actually. Within me.

As we grow our own capacity to self-contain (which means to offer ourselves safety through presence and attention), we understand that feelings don't need soothing. They need and want to simply exist, move, and transform. We align with our own felt experience as women, and we live life oriented by the truth of our yes and no. With self-relating grows the capacity for love and for life to be channeled through these vessels.

It's a lot to live this way. It can sometimes feel like holding live wires. And there are very valid reasons why we are afraid to do so, which we'll explore together.

Since you've picked up this book, I have a feeling you might be walking this path with me. In fact, you may be looking for more ways to express your glorious self and let self-honoring and pleasure be your guide.

If you need permission, legitimization, real and raw reflection, inspiration, and the deep safety that comes from women gathering with intention, I've got you, woman.

Remember, You Know How to Walk in the Dark

Shame is the social regulator that keeps us well-domesticated while driving all of the diagnostic signs and symptoms of disempowerment. It is incredibly expensive, wears a woman down, and keeps her trapped in a too-tight box. Shame coerces you to align with others while your inner little girl cowers, shivering and neglected in the corner of your own heart.

Shame arrests your most vital energy, your *real* power and influence, your sexuality, as well as your erotic wild nature. When you recollect parts of yourself from projections onto others, you learn that being wrong and bad is not, in fact, the same as dying. You learn that the hidden parts of you hold energy that you don't get to enjoy when you are in rejection of self or other. I thoroughly believe we came here to play hide-and-seek with ourselves as conscious embodied beings, to experience *anosognosia*, or to remember what was once known. And it turns out, your responsibility to yourself *is* your responsibility to every single other person on this plane. That's why soul-tending is the most defiant and disruptive changemaking you can engage in. For us all.

So, again, let's get real:

Are you ready to smoke out the shadows and programs that keep you feeling like you're living behind a glass wall?
To compost your dark energy into fertile soil?
To reclaim the creative gifts on the other side of shame?
Unlock the pleasure that's already here?
Drop the mask and feel the lightness of being?
If so, let's do this, beautiful . . .

As we'll explore together, a woman's reclamation journey back home to Self starts with feeling and responding to what I affectionately refer to as her *Fuck No!* Often several, in fact.

This big *No* is an *I EXIST* and *I MATTER* boundary, like when the glaring fluorescent lights pop on in a dimly-lit room. You realize that the people, places, and things you once assumed to be invested in your wellbeing and welfare are not actually as interested as you thought. In psychology, this is called a "rupture of empathy." It's a rupture of trust. It's also the dissolution of an illusion that anchored your former reality. As you reclaim your fierce *No*, you begin to meet your dark feminine parts that hold immense powers (and can be used both for destruction and creation). On the other side of your *No* is desire. It's *Yes*, it's pleasure, it's joy, it's fullness. Ultimately your rupture leads you toward your individuation, your sovereignty, your wholeness, your innate divinity, and your true sense of Self.

Just as so many audacious women have done for me, I'm here to extend my hand to support you as you reclaim your wild woman. As you honor and then dissolve your shamewall. As you crown Your Self.

It's your turn.

Spoiler alert: in order to *woman* (yes, it's a verb to me) as your whole, resourced, womanly self, you first need to mature your inner masculine. And not in the ways you might have thought—no pant-suit, *I'm good, I don't need help*, multitasking, to-do-list-slaying, CEOing.

You must learn how to offer yourself safety.

But first you have to define safety for yourself and understand how it can be sourced, established, and consistently created.

When you aren't offering yourself this kind of containment and instead believe that it's fundamentally up to others to "make" you feel safe, you end up manipulating, strategizing, and micromanaging (and then feel bitter, judgy, and resentful). Which means you ultimately relinquish the opportunity to *feel like a woman*: soft, open, intuiting, and sensing. Instead, you're likely to live in a swirl of confusion that's fueled by the deep knowing of your feminine entitlements, roles, and opportunities that exist in sharp contrast to messages, programs, and a culture that tells you you're doing it plain wrong. This is why most women feel like we're either too much or not enough, too pure or too much of a whore. Mommying too much or working too much. Meanwhile, we feel like everyone is letting us down. No wonder we are tired, wired, and disoriented. But there's a better way, one that you already know deep in your bones. Come on a journey of remembrance with me.

What is a Reclaimed Woman?

I define a Reclaimed Woman as one who is as devoted to herself as to God (insert your preferred term), to her man (and men), to her children (inner and outer), who exudes her heart wisdom and energy in every moment. A Reclaimed Woman is one who feels safe to fully express herself because she knows how to give herself that safety. She knows how to self-husband and set a strong masculine container for her feminine to dance, create, and answer the wild call of her soul— what she actually came here for!

I learned the phrase "self-husband" from my erotic coach, Whitney Lowery, and a caveat may be in order. I am a woman. I have no idea what it is to be a man, to experience reality through the distinct biology of a man's vessel. When I refer to an inner masculine, it is, in most ways, a rhetorical strategy to allow for the identification of certain inner energetic signatures associated with particular thought forms and behaviors. The father introject, or masculine dimension of a woman, is what Carl Jung calls the animus, a projected aspect that we reclaim and integrate through our lived experiences with men.

Because it is my experiential credential, I am speaking to feminine essence women who are confused about how to be a woman. I've walked these grounds myself, and learned that my personality was a mask, that I was living a sweetly well-intentioned lie, that the ways I thought I was keeping myself safe were actually keeping me stuck, and that my essential power was in what I thought was a shameful weakness. We will move through mommy issues, daddy issues, "conspiracy theories," and embodied experiences, ultimately giving you the tools to navigate claiming the gems from your cave, learning what you want and how to ask for it while standing in fierce alignment.

What follows is all about *your* personal reclamation as a woman, designed to help you shed your struggle, choose yourself, and experience the specific pleasure of who you are. My commitment is to lead you home to you.

Woman Up

I'm a big believer in the Maya Angelou quote, "Do the best you can until you know better. Then, when you know better, do better." Part 1 of this book is in service of knowing better, and the rest of the book is about doing better. In Part 1, we'll smoke out the societal shadows that have been keeping us stuck in the throes of victim consciousness. Spoiler alert: it's all by design. At the same time, only *you* hold the keys to free yourself and coronate yourself the Queen of your story. From there, we'll take it into aligned action, which is where your self-initiation officially begins.

Like any good archetypal journey, we'll start with your *No* so that you can find your fully embodied *Yes*.

No

Part 2 is all about your *No*. When you become aware of the fact that you have been self-abandoning, betraying, and rejecting this whole time, imagining it was others doing it to you, you reclaim your power of choice and your capacity to say *No*. But to truly refine this capacity, you must meet all the parts within that you have rejected and welcome them to the table. Your *no way in hell* matures into a *that's not for me, thanks,* and you learn how to play with the darker flavors of your raw erotic essence: your inner Medusa, your inner Kali, your inner dark witch. I like to see your *No* as the combination of your dark feminine inner power that destroys anything less than love, *plus* the light of the matured masculine discernment of a seasoned martial artist who decimates his opponent with nothing more than a glance.

Yes

In Part 3, we move into your *Yes*. Your *Yes* is the light of the feminine: play, creativity, pleasure, receptivity. This is where you tap into your wellspring of creatrix power and get to design your life around your desire and pleasure.

By the end of your heroine's journey, you'll feel excited and curious about challenges and adversity in your life, because you'll know that you came here to dance and play, and that there is nothing more exhilarating than the experience of meeting your full Self. Together we will lay the groundwork for you to recognize and seize all the ripe opportunities you are being presented with to end your suffering. This is a process of discovering and celebrating the polarity within while bringing your inner masculine and feminine into mature, actualized harmony. You'll finally feel like a well-resourced adult, not a secretly flailing child.

Of course, your reclamation experience does not need to look *anything* like mine. You might not pole or twerk in your journey—but also, try it. This is about helping you reconnect to your desire so you can follow that force of attraction wherever it takes you. You'll finally be giving your unhindered inner child a voice, whether she wants to make jewelry, run a farm, wear exquisite hats, live by the ocean, or stay up late giggling with her friends.

One more thing, before we begin—I want you to take a moment and feel the huge field that you are stepping into. The thousands of dogma-defying women who have risen in and through my field, the medical history-making outcomes through my self-care protocol Vital Mind Reset, and the courageous humility that has worn this path so that it can feel softer for your beautiful feet. I attract POWERFUL babes, and you are one of them. HUGE energy is holding your capacity to step out of victimhood and ease into the practice of self-alignment. Feel us all at your back. We've got you, and soon you'll feel that you've got you, no matter what.

And just because it's fun to imagine, offer yourself some audacious "what if's" from where you sit now. I love to open my containers with these prompts, and the responses always bring tears to my eyes because we are remembering, together, to dream into what is possible. So, what if you walked away from chronic illness? What if you healed your relationship with your son? What if you started dancing and became a choreographer? What if you started painting again? *What if?*

PART 1

WOMAN UP

CHAPTER 1

Your Heroine's Journey

Every heroine's journey requires a rite of passage, but the only woman who can initiate you is . . . you.

To embody who you've always been, you *must* self-initiate, then individuate. From there, you self-initiate some more, and then individuate further (it's a rinse and repeat situation). With each cycle, the terrain is more beautiful, and somehow more familiar.

I say "self-initiate" because, due to the hegemony of Western culture, most of us lack societal initiation into our own power. Without rites and rituals to cross over the threshold of adolescence, we carry all of our childhood wounding into adulthood. Instead of maturing with grace, we become children running around in our trauma bodies, masquerading as adults. We maintain well-worn patterns, thoughts, habits, learned ways of being, emotions, and defenses. Sound insane? Welcome to our collective enculturation.

It's up to *you* to walk yourself through your initiatory fire (supported, ideally, by the able hands of women who have walked the path before you) or risk playing the victim for the rest of your life.

The delightful news is that, on your heroine's journey, you get to reclaim your sensuality, your sovereignty, your spine, and—let's face it—your sanity as a woman. Your path of self-devotion asks for a leap of faith. It is worth it, however, because this leap is in service of flight.

I've found that the initiation process is quite archetypal; it's the way to tap into the heroine's journey of lore and legend. In fact, by taking steps forward as a Reclaimed Woman, you are helping to heal our collective community wound and change the way that all women can, well, *woman*.

So let me spin you a yarn as old as time . . .

Once Upon Every Woman's Life

There lived a worn-down miller whose worn-down mill could no longer grind grain into flour, leaving him and his family destitute, though they did the best they could.

One fortuitous day, as the miller made his way home, a mysterious stranger approached with a tempting offer.

"I can make you rich beyond measure—beyond even your wildest fantasies," the stranger cooed. The miller was mesmerized by the velvet in his voice. There was something suspicious about the stranger's offer, but exhausted from years of untold hardship, the miller ignored his own circumspection.

"Surrender everything behind your barn, and I'll bathe you in opulence. You and yours will never want for anything ever again!"

As there was nothing behind the barn but an apple tree, the miller couldn't conjure up a reason to deny the stranger. He wanted the riches, after all, above all.

"Why on earth not?!" He agreed.

Maybe he just got lucky and all will be well!

The bargain struck, the stranger flashed a wicked smile, "I'll come back in three years' time to claim what's mine," and he vanished.

No sooner had he left than the miller's wife, bedecked in finery and dripping jewels, ran into his embrace, marveling at their change in fortune.

"It's a miracle! How did this happen?" his delighted wife cried.

The miller explained his bargain: all the wealth and riches they'd ever need, for the small price of everything behind the barn.

Instantly, his wife's face lost all its sparkle and color, a stark contrast to her silks and gems.

"Husband, how could you forget? Our daughter is always behind the barn at this time, sweeping the yard with her willow broom." Her shoulders dropped, softly she repeated, "Husband, how could you forget?"

And just like that, the miller realized his folly; in his exhaustion and greed, he had offered up his beloved daughter to the devil.

Over the next three years, surrounded by constant lavish reminders of the price they'd paid, the young woman blossomed into young adulthood, maintaining an aura of innocence and purity even as she waited for the devil to claim her.

Three years to the day, the dutiful maiden washed and readied herself in a simple white dress, then drew a salt circle around herself in anticipation of the devil's arrival. When he appeared, she held her head high, even though her hands were shaking. He grabbed at her, but his hands couldn't penetrate the boundary of the salt circle; he was repelled across the yard. In forceful anger, he tried again to claim her for himself, but once again he was rebuffed. She was mysteriously untouchable.

"She's too pure," the devil surmised. "The next time I come, she must be tarnished. Don't let her bathe."

When the devil returned, the maiden was covered in grime, ripe with her own body's odors, hair tangled and nails foul with filth, while her parents looked on with shame.

Upon seeing the devil again, the maiden wept, large gulping sobs with fat cleansing tears that washed her filth away—leaving her too clean for the devil, whose grasping hands were once again deflected by her purity.

Enraged, the devil gave them one last chance.

"Chop off her hands."

Seeing the miller about to protest, he added "Or I'll kill you all. You have three days."

The miller was horrified, and his wife broke down in a heap: defeated, lost, paralyzed. Their daughter remained brave. "Do it, father." She offered her hands up and laid them on the chopping block. "I am your child, and I trust you."

Out of fear of the devil, and before he could lose his nerve, her father did the unthinkable—he lifted his axe high and chopped off his daughter's hands.

As her perfectly pure hands hit the ground, both father and daughter wailed, a scream that tore through them both for the horrible fortune that had brought them to this grim tableau.

From this moment on, the girl was no longer who she had been.

When the devil returned, he found her handless, but nevertheless clean from her own purifying tears of anguish. He realized, finally, that he could never lay hands on the young maiden, so he relinquished his claim and vanished back into the recesses of the forest.

The family kept their hollow riches and decided to move to town to start anew, but the daughter chose not to accompany them. She no longer felt she belonged, and she had no interest in the luxury her father had to offer, her stumps an endlessly bitter reminder of the price they paid for a lavish life.

"I will go to the forest."

Her mother bandaged her hands in silence as her father watched; words were pointless, for she had let go of everything she knew, and everything she'd once been.

To be continued . . .

This is the start to "The Handless Maiden," a folktale that's been handed down across generations and cultures, recounted by the Brothers Grimm, and stunningly rendered by Dr. Clarissa Pinkola Estés in *Women Who Run With the Wolves*. Estés encourages us to view folktales as holofractal experiences, each character essentially representing a part of the woman's psyche. As such, we can see the miller as the immature masculine dimension of ourselves: the father-wounded woman, who trades away her inner kingdom for quick fixes that all too soon prove devastating. Estés details that "The Handless Maiden" is one of many folktales that starts with a father betraying his daughter, exchanging her life force for a shot at a so-called "easier" and richer life. The miller represents the part of us that strikes a poor bargain with life: "When a woman surrenders her instincts that tell her the right time to say yes and when to say no, when she gives up her insight, intuition, and other wildish traits, then she finds herself in situations that promised gold but ultimately give grief."[1]

This is the *poor bargain*.

The betrayal the maiden experiences at the hands of her father is her very first rupture of empathy. This act of (self-)betrayal catalyzes the long initiatory journey back home to Self. Estés illuminates:

> [T]he poor bargain, like birth and death, constitutes a rather utilitarian step off the cliff planned by the Self in order to bring a woman deep into her wildness. A woman's initiation begins with the poor bargain she made long ago while still slumbering . . . That female psychic slumber is a state approximating somnambulism. During it, we walk, we talk, yet we are asleep. We love, we work, but our choices tell the truth about our condition; the voluptuous, the inquiring, the good and incendiary sides of our natures are not fully sentient.[2]

So how does this translate for women today?

I would venture to argue that, at one point or another, you've made a poor bargain too . . .

Essentially, the poor bargain is a choice to exchange suppression of your own awareness for seeming security, convenience, or power. When you "play it safe" and subsist on the crumbs of life, you accept the poor bargain. When you take the bait of a too-good-to-be-true solution, you accept the poor bargain. When you fail to trust that you always have all that you need to walk your specific path in life, you accept the poor bargain, and you will continue to do so until you decide to say *Yes* to your initiatory invitation. The decision-making apparatus of your personality strikes survival-based bargains that seem to yield returns early in childhood, but those same bargains cost you dearly later in life. Your inner parts stop talking to each other and, often, one inner protector takes the wheel and decides that

7

social acceptance, quick fixes, or tolerating and ignoring red flags is worth it, as other parts protest and clamor in the background.

In childhood, love and attention are core needs; you cannot survive without them. To fulfill these needs, you learn to curate the aspects of yourself that are most likely to give you love, and you learn to hide the parts of yourself that might be seen as raw, wild, bad, or otherwise punishable by withdrawal of affection, or worse.

The maiden's refusal to live with her parents after experiencing this betrayal is her big *Fuck No* to life as she knew it. Her rite of passage is brought about by deep wounding (in every sense of the word), so she goes off into the forest on a vision quest and begins her process of self-initiation.

It's time we uncover the collective poor bargain that we, as women, make—pretty much every damn day of our lives until we're ready to find our *No*, burn shit down, and reclaim our full, wild, selves.

It all starts with a concerted assault on human wildness.

The War on Eros

One of the most pervasive agendas shaping the collective is the war against the fundamentally erotic nature of this incarnation—*we came from sex after all!*—and the resultant warfare against the body, between men and women, and the objectification of sexuality as something that we can use, acquire, and leverage. In fact, it's my humble opinion that the attack on eros is something that's many decades, if not centuries, in the making.

So, what is eros, exactly?

Eros is your animating life force (also known as "chi," "prana," or "vital force energy"). It is the aliveness that flows when there are no constrictions and contractions: your intuitive guidance, your felt sense of *Yes* and *No* in your body. Eros is self-propagating and regenerating: a cup of embodied love that's always full. It is your soul's authentic song, what makes up the fabric of *you*. Moving up from Mother Earth, eros flows through the energetic channels of your cervix, heart, throat, crown, and back down to her in what is often referred to as a "microcosmic orbit." The flow of this life force energy lives within us, moves between us, and weaves us into the fabric of nature. Eros expresses creatively, and she cannot, will not, be programmed (sorry AI). It's the expression of a divine impulse through the sensory technology of your physical vessel.

Eros is your birthright. When you awaken to your eros, you get to delight in the understanding, knowing, and feeling that you and your body are on the same team and that the messages (i.e., symptoms), sensations, and expressions from your body matter. From there, your body becomes a channel for life force. Life force is *creative* as in pro-creative or creating *life*, but also in creating ideas, things, explorations, movements, and visions.

Unfortunately, we've been conditioned to normalize disconnection from this vital force energy and encouraged to gaslight ourselves into being "okay" when this disconnection should feel anything but. Psychiatrists like Dr. Alexander Lowen, who wrote *Fear of Life*, help us to understand some of the early roots of this disconnection through Oedipal psychology and the triangulation of young children with their parents when they are raised without a larger community (which is most of us).[3]

As we become aware of our own eros, so, too, do our parents. As daughters, we enter into a dynamic with our fathers, and into tension with our mothers. It is said that girls develop a fear that their erotic energy (which is expressed as prancing across a room, singing, laughing, "showing off," tantrums, or more recognizably self-pleasuring) could get them punished or rejected to the point of existential threat if it is misplaced, unwelcome, or even incompletely available. Women afraid of their own erotic energy might choose to partner with "nice guy" males, compete with and disrespect the alpha men they fear, condemn other women for expressing their sexuality, or use their sexual energy to manipulate and seduce men as a personal security strategy.

9

Sons, on the other hand, develop a fear of castration by their "shadow mommies," who are conflicted about their own relationship to the masculine, healthy aggression, and male sexuality; these mothers can take on these boys as subdued spousal surrogates or parentified children. The castration effect yields mommy-pleasers whose energy has been stuffed into a shame-encased container. Boys suffer what River Roaring calls "boner shame," where they are humiliated by any experience of arousal or penile movement but then later expected to have rock-hard cocks in the bedroom for the duration of any lovemaking session.

We want the wolf, but we raise the lamb.

This is how men and women, alike, land themselves in the trauma space of punishment and shame tied to sexual embodiment. We are so disconnected from our own inner drives, ignorant of the ways in which our sexuality is operating from behind the curtain of our shame, that we project our disavowed parts onto other women (judging, at turns, both the Madonna and the whore) and onto men as being perpetrators against our innocence. Women start telling other women how they "should" dress and act, and sexuality becomes something that *happens* rather than an energy to be channeled. It is objectified by both men and women rather than integrated and energetically mastered.

The first step in this self-mastery journey is growing the capacity to be with the energy of shame. Like a phantom, shame guards all the things you were told you're not allowed to be, feel, or do. Every time you feel bad and wrong (and let's face it, most women have been trained to believe there is something fundamentally wrong with them) a bit of your eros gets trapped behind what I call a *shamewall*. You lose access to your most vital force, and you source dregs from a small percentage of the infinite energy that could be at your disposal. Your light is dimmed, and the people around you can feel and sense where you have deadened, stiffened, and are otherwise pretending to be all there.

When your sexual energy is shamed into a catacomb (from simple admonishments like "stop jumping on the couch!" to punishment for self-pleasure), it can feel like you're completely cut off from life, your inner drive and guidance, and that you require others to tell you how to be you. It feels like answers live outside of you, and you are trapped in the victim consciousness that keeps you at the feet of those outside forces.

We've all been there.

I've come to understand that you're only as free as your darkest secret. And most of our secret chambers are home to tales of body shame, sexual repression and objectification, and a motley crew of "never do or be that in public." Our conditioning is so deep, at this point, that it's almost hard to recognize how divorced we are from our own sensuality and our own sexuality . . . from our *aliveness*. We distract ourselves by imagining that this is a war between free civilians and government, natural medicine and allopathy, liberals and conservatives . . . but *this is a war between the energy of sovereign human vitalism and dehumanizing parasitism.* Yes, it's the power of the embodied human against those forces that feed off of human emotion—chiefly fear—to enslave and control humanity as a perpetual source of vital force energy.

We've been programmed to believe that our inherent nature as women (soft and messy; creative and sensual; hungry, full, and wanting more) is fundamentally inappropriate, harmful to others, or too dangerous to express, which means that shutting down is a wise strategy. When we are disconnected from our eros, we are left to feel totally divorced from our bodies, and we are much more likely to recruit parentified systems (like the allopathic industrial medical complex and big daddy government) to "save us," causing us to fight against our authentic selves rather than rise up and own ourselves. That's how victim consciousness works. It's all about recruiting an outside authority to help you fix the thing that you think is broken (about you).

This is why our collective poor bargain seemed like such a good deal, at the time. *Just don't look at the devil behind the curtain!*

Your Poor Bargain

Subjected to three waves of feminism, women today have suffered a tremendous bait and switch: the false promise that when we prove we can do everything men do—*while* bleeding (i.e., during the placebo week of our birth control pills)—we'll finally feel fulfilled, fed, and fired up by life.

We've become over-caffeinated CEOs, haggard single moms, and overachieving, under-touched "boss-babes," who imagine that intimacy looks like wine and Netflix (but without any chill). We are bitter, resentful, and disappointed. Most. Of. The. Time. And we have all sorts of theories about how right we are about how wronged we've been.

We strive toward an impossible paradox every day: Be strong enough to rise and thrive, but also soft enough to hold a baby safely in your arms. Be beautiful and perfectly poised in public but be a lusty love bunny behind closed doors. Nurture everyone—except yourself. This duality leads to feelings of shame, incompleteness, and sometimes total self-abandonment, which leads to a life where we settle for getting what we don't want, and we pretend we're "fine" when we don't get what we *do* want.

Enculturated Good Girls, we cringe at the idea of being called "selfish" while venerating "selflessness" as proof of worth. There's a hollowness to our life experiences, even in the moments that "should" feel spectacular. I liken that hollowness to living behind a glass wall and believe this experience to be a surefire diagnostic sign for the poor bargain.

The good news is that taking the poor bargain might have been your soul's design to re-acquaint you with your wildness. Because if you choose to accept your audacious mission, your self-abandonment will lead you to your *Fuck No* so that you can find your *Fuck Yes*.

And since we do better when we know better, we need to talk about the greatest psyop women have ever faced. The poorest bargain of them all. And that, lovely human, is feminism.

CHAPTER 2

Feminism: The Greatest Bait & Switch of All Time

A woman's highest calling is to lead a man to his soul, so as to unite him with Source . . . A man's highest calling is to protect a woman, so she is free to walk the earth unharmed.

—Cherokee Proverb

There's no winning the war between men and women when we are pitted against one another, and it is my firm belief that the political movement called feminism has baited women into fighting for empowerment at the expense of men, leaving us exhausted, bitter, and resentful.

The feminist movement promised that we would get ours, that we would know freedom and power, and that we would no longer suffer what it is to be a woman. We were promised freedom from our roles in the household, our reproductive imperative, and even from the constraints of a female body. Sexuality was rendered a recreational activity to be infused with whatever meaning you assign it, no different from any other social interaction. As we deny the biological reality of a woman's roles and vulnerabilities, we also deny the reality that women live in a world with men. And we strike a poor bargain when our sexual freedom is contingent upon our sexual appeal, which is a very limited game for women to play over the course of our lifetimes. A game that denies the root power of a woman's energetic and erotic gifts, whether she's making love, giving a lecture, or stirring a pot of soup.

We have been led to believe that since men have historically held the power, they've dominated and abused us. And now that we are rising up, it's their turn to pay, and they better run. But do we *really* want men to apologize, cower, and appease us? Do we really even want what they have? And what is it that they have, exactly?

For most of human history, men have led merciless lives. War, suicide, violence, extraordinarily dangerous jobs: these are the statistical realities that define the male experience. Perhaps a very small percentage of men represent those "in control," but the underdogs are certainly on both sides of the aisle of sexes. You won't hear me use the word "patriarchy" to throw a barb at the men I hold responsible for my un-stewarded vulnerability. Patriarchy is about power dynamics and zero-sum games, not men. Perhaps we are really looking to blame and shame the bad daddy, rather than men as an axiomatic faction of society—but more on father woundology later.

Both men and women have experienced unique and intersecting struggles. If I were to sum up the plight of all women across all time, it might come down to *unsafety*.

A woman's biology is designed to create and nurture life, and so she is the blooming bud, the flickering flame, the drop of water that yearns for sacred attention, protection, and containment. She is, by her very nature, vulnerable. By allowing ourselves to be colonized by the hegemony of masculine values, we have abdicated intimacy with what is valuable to us as women, gaslighting ourselves into thinking that achievement, success, and productivity are the keys to fulfillment.

So, a few quick questions:

Are we really looking to gain status and power in the marketplace so that we can imitate the men we are fundamentally afraid of? Isn't that like dressing up as a monster on Halloween?

Is safety found in forty+ hour work weeks, separation from our children, neglect of our bodies, competition with our sisters, tension with our partners, and endless consumerism?

Or:

Does safety stem from restoring connections with biology, with nature, with each other, and the prioritization of our own erotic energy, and from the invitation for men to step into purpose, providership, and protectorship?

If the latter is true, perhaps it is not power *over men* that we seek, but the restoration of the truly empowered man, so that we can finally exhale and get back to what we do best: feel, create, intuit, and channel.

Reclaiming our sense of balance requires that we acknowledge a root cause of our oppression, which is the denial of our very real and sacred vulnerability as women, as well as the existential terror of being in a woman's body. Maybe you don't care about a harmonious, expansive romantic union where you and your man are on the same team, navigating the balance of autonomy and connection together. Maybe you have other problems to focus on or have cast all men into the reject pile. The thing is, whether you have sex with them or won't ever, *you walk in a world with men.* Acknowledging that most men can kill any woman, any time they please, shines light on how we relate to sex and sexuality, and the bait we might take when offered socially-engineered prospects of feminism and sexual liberation. On the other hand, denying this reality leads to all sorts of manipulation, strategy, and bargaining for safety.

How Did We Get Into This Mess?

You're welcome, ladies. Because of the good fight fought, you get to don your pantsuit, pay taxes, and be a corporate baddie sharing the provider role with a man while still managing the majority of the domestic workload and all the invisible labor that women contribute. Apparently, some women still believe that we are in a better place bracing ourselves against the men we choose to marry, establishing our independence, bringing monetary value to the table, controlling as many decisions as possible in the home, and fundamentally diminishing his role, purpose, importance, and incentive to actualize his mission. This dynamic often leads to terrible romantic relationships, with 70 percent of divorces currently initiated by unhappy wives. In fact, I can count on one hand, or maybe even two fingers, how many *healthy erotic partnerships* I know.

Has it always been like this? Men and women, oil and water? Perhaps it's meant to be like this, perhaps this war is just one of many wars that come with the resonance field of victim consciousness. According to many, "the feminist movement" was a Rockefeller-funded, socially engineered political movement primarily intended to offer women the poison apple of egalitarian opportunity while removing them and their children from the home.

A word on social engineering so as to dispel any suspicion that mass movements simply "occur." In fact, for the better part of a hundred years, the collective unconscious has been strategically manipulated through coordinated efforts between the CIA and the Tavistock Institute for Human Relations, which is "the psychological warfare arm of the British Royal family . . . the world's most important institution for the manipulation of population."[1] With tentacles in the psychedelic, New Age, sexual liberation, feminist, aliens, trans and more "movements," media and entertainment are controlled by some of the most adept psychological researchers on this plane (did you know that the Tavistock Institute created MTV and that the Pentagon has a film budget?!). And we are available for hypnosis because we have not yet reclaimed ourselves. As Freud wrote in *Mass Psychology*, "The mass has never thirsted for truth, they demand illusions and cannot do without them."[2] When we are dispossessed of our emotions and lack the self-mastery of adult consciousness, we are susceptible to poor bargains, manipulation, and groupthink. We let ourselves go in hopes of belonging; consciously or unconsciously, we sell our souls.

Anyway, the feminist movement extracted us from the role as the primary caretaker of our children, rendered us additional taxpayers, and created the conditions for industrialized schooling to program children into good workers. Over time, we became more and more disconnected from our role as nurturers, our reverence for the natural world, our cyclical nature, and our intuition. We became embittered corporate climbers, in competition with men *and* with women.

Here's what women have come to believe:

- Women have suffered and are now entitled
- Women should act strong and independent
- Women know better how to do things
- Women should hide their sexual energy unless they want to invite harm
- There are sluts and there are respectable women
- Men and women are the same
- Men owe women
- Men are stupid, violent, and savage
- Men only want to take sex and can't control their sexual impulses
- Men who don't acknowledge a woman's sexuality are respecting them

This narrative goes so far as to insist that we have virtually no need for men any longer other than for occasional sexual recreation. Really? I'm pretty sure that I'd have no house to live in, lights to turn on, water to wash with, car to drive, or computer to type on without them, for starters. I've found, anecdotally, that women who are steeped in that psychology, whether in a relationship or not, are some of the least ecstatic, least vibrant, least fulfilled, and most righteously bitter humans on the face of the plane. As a woman, I have a yearning to live in a safe(r) world where men rise to their most honorable and valiant expression, and honor and protect the women and children of the collective. I believe that both men's and women's nervous systems require the assurance of *many* strong men at our backs. The route to this nirvana may be more in my control, as a woman, than I formerly imagined, as it may be for you. And it may have everything to do with how we interact with men in our lives, relate to sex, motherhood, and the institution of marriage. But first, we must jailbreak from feminist psychology.

To add to the dizzying blurring of sex roles, natural contracts, vulnerabilities, and responsibilities, we have the Jung-inspired and Tavistock-leveraged New Age movement in which we have been encouraged to transcend the limitations of our bodies. Men have been encouraged to cry and emote with women, to rise above their anger, and to let go of outdated constructs like masculine providership and protectorship. Long-haired, flowy, yoga practicing, free spirits, New Age men are a far cry from the chicken bone ripping, rapey, warrior brothers of yore. But thanks to all of these agendas, women and men are meeting somewhere in the gender-neutralized egalitarian middle. Meanwhile polarity, eros, and healthy marriage are suffering, as is the family unit and our understanding of parental roles and responsibilities. To turn the females in a species against their reproductive imperative, against the monogamous pairings that serve and protect those roles, and in support of hook-up culture and the minimization of the inherent meaning of sex, is a feat of epic proportions.

The required cognitive dissonance is immense.

As is the gaslighting of women who are told that they should feel empowered and free when they are mimicking men in society, self- and pharmaceutically medicating all the ways in which their body, mind, and spirit are saying no (ways that are pathologized into diagnoses like anxiety, ADHD, and depression). Philosopher Jiddu Krishnamurti reportedly said, "It's no sign of health to be well-adapted to a profoundly sick society," but women are told that they should feel well, happy, and fulfilled while disconnected from the natural world, their cycles, their children, their food, and the men in the world. This feat would be nearly impossible if not for the foot soldiers of the feminist agenda: birth control and psychotropic medications, specifically antidepressants. Designed to feel, women had to be disconnected from themselves through some heavy chemical artillery, positioning us as helpless victims who can be more easily subdued by top-down, socioculturally normalized interventions. When we have been persuaded that we, as women, are victimized by our own female biology and psychoemotional nature, we beg to be relieved of it by an outside authority.

I know because I was one of these women who proudly took birth control for twelve years leading up to my Hashimoto's diagnosis and specialized in defending the right to meds for women of reproductive age. Consisting of synthetic hormones that can chemically sterilize and hormonally hijack women, more than contraception is achieved with birth control; deeper connection to our energetic power is blocked. And when these women experience the known effects of birth control pills, rings, and injections, including mood and cognitive symptoms, they are dismissed and told that "it's all in their head," which leads them where? To the shrink! Who then offers psychotropic medications for depression, anxiety, insomnia, and even mania and psychotic symptoms which then have their own spiritual, psychological, and physical effects driving further medications and diagnoses. A "sick" identity is crystalized, and another God channel captured.

Here's how it goes:

A woman's body wisely responds to a nutrient-deficient, inflammatory diet, toxicant body burden, draining zero-sum game relationships, her unacknowledged trauma patterns, and the collapsing of her spiral energy into the linear path of performance that corporate expectations dictate. She is told that her body's wise response to these stressors represents a pathology: hormonal imbalance or PCOS (polycystic ovary syndrome) or PMS or luteal insufficiency, and she is prescribed a ring, pills, or injected birth control.

Her thyroid, sex, and stress hormones hijacked, she is no longer ovulating or experiencing her body's rhythmic feedback, but now she has bigger issues. Her mood is erratic, she hasn't been sleeping, she's gained weight, she has brain fog, and her libido is an afterthought. Her prescriber dismisses her and sends her to a friendly psychiatrist

19

who prescribes an antidepressant. In a few weeks, she goes off the rails with irritability and insomnia and is told she now has bipolar disorder; she is prescribed an antipsychotic and a mood stabilizer.

Fast forward twenty-five years and she's on five meds, a hollow shell of herself with a laundry list of diagnoses, and she's told to just keep being a good patient.

As a reproductive psychiatrist who spent a decade in the trenches, I've exposed the medical literature condemning synthetic birth control as poison that leads to more poison. I've also published my own medical literature that proves even the most extreme premenstrual dysphoria can be reversed through lifestyle change—within two cycles! It's my belief that psychiatric medications are the most habit-forming chemicals on this plane. And this is not to mention the gross underreporting of known adverse effects, including impulsive acts of suicide and violence, and the overpromising of so-called efficacy.

These medications, whether by design or unintended consequence, further entrench the fragmentation of parts that drive problematic behavior and painful patterns of experience. Your witness consciousness and inner awareness go offline, and your feeling parts are locked more deeply into the closet, while numb protector parts are brought to the fore. They arrest the development and maturation of the ensouled being, and they pit you against you as you wake up daily to your name on the label of that pill bottle, conditioning yourself further into the belief that *something is wrong with you*. Thank goodness for the savior that is the medical system! It boils down to a simple vector of allegiance:

A woman says *No* to her body when she says *Yes* to Pharma.

Many neoliberal feminist pundits don't like when I say this. In fact, I received aerial shots of my house with death threats from a feminist media outlet (Pharma subsidized) in 2016 after writing an article on homebirth that inspired waves of trolls to mount a campaign characterizing me as an "ableist" (a slur in the eugenics family, it appears). Well, when I wore the "ableist" Villain Crown, I found it to have some truth glimmering from the spikes and snarls atop my head. I *do* believe that any woman—and I mean *any* woman—can reclaim herself from the grips of agendas that have her hypnotized. She is able to birth a baby in bliss at home, she is able to mature into self-care, right lifestyle choices, and emotional self-mastery, she is able to walk away from diagnoses and prescriptions, and she is able to find safety in herself and her relationships without the help of man-shaming and hate programming.

There is a better way, but it requires the audacity to take radical responsibility for your own health and to say *Yes* to the wisdom of your biology.

The Dupe of the Sexual Revolution

In *The Case Against the Sexual Revolution*, Louise Perry declares that "the prescription [of freedom] doesn't cure the disease."[3] And that, dear reader, is the plight of the modern woman in a nutshell. Perhaps it wasn't ever freedom that we were after. Perhaps, as David Deida teaches, freedom is the striving of the masculine, while love is the yearning of the feminine.

Perry does an excellent job of describing how it is that we came to demand the wrong medicine for the struggles of the 1960s woman. If we are looking to make poor bargains, then it certainly makes sense that "having what he's having" might seem like a viable solution to the problem of being a woman in a domineering man-led society. If a woman is surrounded by men who are not taking her best interest as their own, she might imagine that imitating those men would confer power and status to her life. The freedom to be more like men in the world is like taking a Tylenol for a piece of glass stuck in your foot; the root cause of the problem is neglected by the proposed solution. This "solution," in turn, destroys the infrastructure of family, marriage, and motherhood that sustains a woman's personal fulfillment, even if she ultimately chooses to work in a way that can be woven in and through these natural priorities. When a woman's natural gifts and talents are commodified, however, she becomes someone who offers nurturance, creativity, and care to strangers, for hire, rather than to her own husband, children, and family.

Perry sums it up:

> *The atomised worker with no commitment to any place or person is the worker best able to respond quickly to the demands of the market. This ideal liberal subject can move to wherever the jobs are because she has no connection to anywhere in particular; she can do whatever labour is asked of her without any moral objection derived from faith or tradition; and, without a spouse or family to attend to, she never needs to demand rest days or a flexible schedule. And then, with the money earned from this rootless labour, she is able to buy consumables that will soothe any feelings of unhappiness, thus feeding the economic engine with maximum efficiency.*[4]

Thanks to the sexual liberation movement and its henchmen—birth control, medicalized birth, formula feeding, and antidepressants—we women can be cogs in the capitalistic wheel just like men, and we can also "fuck like men," disabused of our species stewardship. But is no-strings-attached sex really what we want, as women? Perry argues that although we've been encouraged to be callous about sexual experiences and social interaction, it *does*, in fact, matter to women. To *pretend* that sex is not important to women is a gaslight. Perry suggests that we behave as though we do, in fact, have a deep feeling that sex is special. If we didn't, rape would be no different than any form of violence, and sexual harassment would be no different than bullying. She writes:

> *The liberal feminist argument leads us to conclude that, if you are going to destroy the sexual double standard, then you must use your own body, and the bodies of other women, as a battering ram against the patriarchal edifice. The advice to young women*

is that you must 'fuck back' if you want to be a good feminist, and mostly it will turn out OK—and when it doesn't? When a sexual encounter turns out to be 'not-ideal', or worse? Well then, we must fall back on liberal feminism's old standby: 'teach men not to rape.'[5]

Perry identifies that when we pretend that sexual appetites and consequences are the same for men and women, we ignore the reality of pregnancy, and we also ignore a body of published literature on what's called sociosexuality, which very clearly demonstrates that men have more diversified sexual interests than women, who prefer monogamous pairings. And this difference is, dear reader, because men and women are, indeed, different. So, is it any wonder that the veneration of masculinized casual sex has left so many of us epically confused about our sexuality and how best to live in accordance with our biology?

Women's True Power

What if our true power is to be gatekeepers and guardians of our own sexual energy, and we've taken yet another poor bargain imagining that power would arise from the gaslight that says we can have sex that's just for fun. What if restricting access to sex to men who are father-ready providers is the real play? I suspect that this self-valuing behavior on the part of women may very well inspire more father-ready providers. Said another way, recognizing sex as sacred makes the world safer for women.

If we women only offered our sexuality to men who would make good providers and fathers, it might be dismissed as practicing hypergamy, being "trad wives," or fishing for men of higher status, but we may actually be restoring a system that *works* for women and men. The biological reality is that for both men and women, the mastery of one's sexual impulses and discernment around when to express and suppress them is a huge part of what makes the world safer for women. This safer world recognizes that women can only be women when our basic needs are cared for.

So, you want to run a seven-figure business as a girl boss? Here's a telegram from the trenches: It's definitely possible, but I can't *imagine* how much easier and more delightful it would be to live my CEO dreams if I didn't have to experience the pressure of making what I call "masculine money" to keep the lights on for my kids and make a long list of payments while enjoying my opportunity to play the capitalist game. If I were provided for by a male breadwinner, I'd be truly liberated to make *feminine* money, to allow my playful impulses free reign, and to expand the creative—erotic—energy field in the world without the constraint of survival stress. My soul might enjoy a long-sought-after exhale. This exhale is designed to be offered to women in a society of initiated men, incentivized to get their maturational shit together by the prospect of wife-ing a high value woman.

I hear the objections from the back of the room:

"But I 'have to' bring money home or we wouldn't be able to pay the bills."

"But there just aren't good successful men out there."

"But I have higher earning potential than my husband."

"But that's just not realistic because I'd be dependent and vulnerable if I stopped earning . . . "

And here's how I respond to those objections: Thanks to the swing of the pendulum toward women masculinizing, you can earn what you want, and you don't need to be with a man. So don't choose one who isn't qualified to provide and then complain about it. That's called trying to buy eggs from the hardware store.

Don't choose a man that you don't fundamentally trust and respect. Just don't do it (I'll offer my support with this in Part 3). Because you *do* have a choice, and partnering erotically or maritally should be from the deep desire to belong to that man and for him to belong to you, both of you devoted to God or something greater than the two of you. It's easier to choose a good man when you do not open yourself to creating life with someone who would not be a good provider or father. So, exercise your power of choice and discernment when it comes to offering yourself to men erotically. For every woman who does this, we move forward into the land of restoration and reclamation of the sexes as they are designed to synergize.

From what I can tell, no feminist ideology addresses the imperative to restore the contracts that men and women incarnated to uphold. How do we move beyond fear of men who do not take women's wellbeing as their own, and into harmony and complementarity?

I believe that our power lies in three specific arenas that translate into systemic safety, collective change, and the kind of feminine impulses that serve our sisters and our children. The first is the reclamation of courtship as the gatekeeping of our erotic energy based on the accurate assessment of safety (we'll be learning how to assess safety in Part 2!). The second is the reclamation of the covenant of marriage and specifically the way that we as women can choose to get in our lane and align with our stated desires to experience the power of the man that we have chosen and to end cycles of mother-son dynamics in romantic relationships that don't serve husbands or wives (more in Part 3). Third is what I would call the sovereign mothering of sons. Though I don't have a son and don't have direct experience in this arena, I do know that this is one of the systemic roots of the unsafe world that we live in as women. I believe that as women walk themselves home through the self-relating tools outlined in this book, we will no longer mother sons from the shadow realms of our fear. Women will no longer castrate their boys energetically and demand that they regulate their mother's emotional systems, and boys will learn healthy aggression and how to have intimacy with their darkness. As Jordan Peterson often relates, you can't trust a man unless you know that he can kill and is choosing not to, and we can contribute to growing this population of trustworthy men, directly.

Through these efforts on our part, men will grow to self-tame, to self-initiate, and to come into brotherhood again. This is what it will take to bring their hearts and spines back online and to restore the union of the sexes that I know in my heart is possible.

The other day, my beloved handyman was telling me that his son is considering becoming a welder because of how well it pays. We spoke about how dangerous and demanding the job apparently is, and I said, "You know, I look around sometimes at all the stuff. Literally, all of it—the buildings, the roads, the infrastructure of our society, and I recognize that men did all of that dangerous, back-breaking labor. I think about the literal team of men I've employed, as a single woman, to fix everything that breaks, and I'm so appreciative."

He replied, "We do it all for you."

Perhaps that's the contract in a nutshell; a woman inspires providership, service, and protectorship by simply existing, and her appreciation closes the circuit on the most powerful free-energy device there is: the man-woman polarity.

As We Heal Within, Man-Woman Relating Evolves

This "power" that women have achieved is like a lick of ice cream when we really want a tall glass of water. True feminine power is heart wisdom, the fullness that always wants more, and the destruction of "anything less than love," as David Deida would say. It is the churning, moving, alchemical cauldron of endless creation. Desire is a woman's compass, and feelings are the weather by which she navigates.

In his rubric of feminine and masculine energetic dynamics, Deida describes the process of maturing through three stages. It begins with manipulative, fear-based taking from relationships, then evolves into the negotiation of transactional need-meeting and ends in devotional service between man and woman as channels of divine energy.[6]

Through one lens, feminism and sexual liberation served to *masculinize women (animus-possess)* and the New Age to *feminize men (anima-possess)*. But when we resist the activist stance that says *Look at what those puppet masters did, socially engineering our disempowerment,* we are reminded that there are no mistakes and that the capacity to hold the tension of opposites is a marker of adult psychology. So yes, we've been duped. We devoured the poison apple with gusto, *and* everything is exactly as it needs to be for our collective and individual actualization. Perhaps this neutralization of the sexes and the resultant cold war that's resulted in abysmal divorce rates, with one in four women on an antidepressant, and a climate of "us against them," is *exactly what we needed* to progress from the first-stage version of man-woman dynamics into the more balanced, individuated second stage. We needed, as women, to reclaim the animus, to recognize the light and dark aspects of the masculine within, in order to choose to align with our feminine nature.

Deida also describes how a helpless, desperate, manipulative first-stage woman then becomes self-sufficient in her second stage and helps herself. Then in the third stage, she reconnects to her heart's yearning to be helped, protected, and provided for by a man as devoted to her as he is to God, and she chooses to artfully express that authentic vulnerability in service of the sacred contract between woman and man. Developing these third-stage dynamics requires the surrender of much of the societally conditioned defensive structure that has been adopted for self-protection and survival. Deida calls these "shells," which can present in many ways, such as a woman who becomes intellectually identified and thus strives to be recognized for what she does, rather than who she is. She then goes on to attract a feminized man who thinks he wants an independent woman, but who really, deep down, wants a devoted submissive to support him. While she thinks she wants a feeling-centered man, at her essence she really wants a dominant alpha to fend for her.

This courageous, dominant man can offer attentive attunement that stabilizes a woman's nervous system, allowing her energy to flow into and through him. This segregation of roles and vectorization of energies is referred to as polarity. And Deida would say that you can recognize if you are wired as a feminine essence being if you long to be *ravished*. Not raped in heart-disconnected dominance, but fervently,

27

enthusiastically, and sensually taken, while the one who feels the drive to ravish and penetrate is in the masculine essence polarity.[7]

> *It is one of the contradictions of life that a flow has to be contained to maintain its movement.*
> —Alexander Lowen, MD, *Fear of Life*[8]

Although women have held their tongues on the inherent differences between men and women (likely due to cancel culture), the collective feminine desire to be ravished is alive and well. This desire was never made so clear to me as when I presented at the Weston A. Price conference in 2022. During the Q&A, I responded to a question about gender dynamics with the statement, "Most women I know long to be well-handled by a powerful man," and a sensual sigh—an ecstatic swoon—swept across the two-thousand-person room. This experience felt like permission to acknowledge our deeply-held desire to exhale, stop the hypervigilance, the multitasking, and the full-on pretending that true feminine fulfillment could *ever* be found at the top of a corporate ladder.

Through courageous self- and other-relating, we now have the opportunity to peel back the layers of programming and self-protection, find our heart's longing, and take steps in the direction of divine union, ecstatic sexual embodiment, and inner and outer polarity.

So, how does a woman become a match for this ravishment experience once she has practiced honoring her body, emotions, and needs the way she longs for a man to?

She gets in her lane.

Her lane is to be the pulsing, beating heart of the relationship, sensing what needs to be expressed in real time. Whether this is a pouty "ouch" or a dagger-filled glare or spontaneous tears, Deida teaches about the power of residue-less emotion that is expressed with an open heart in the moment.

A woman's lane is also to offer respect, appreciation, and the guardianship of her man's reputation—and to only partner with men she can authentically offer this to.

I, like many women, experienced an immediate rupture in the man-woman contract when I have been with a man who is defensive, dismissive, takes the emotional microphone, cries, emotes, and is otherwise volatile rather than self-possessed, regulated, grounded, and outwardly attuned in the presence of women and children. Because I cannot offer respect to a man who is emotionally dispossessed, I cannot expect him to naturally meet my needs for safety and containment in return. Persisting in this dynamic is a recipe for contempt and the repatterning of eggs-from-the-hardware-store impossible love.

Expressed Polarity

In a healthy romantic dyad, feminine and masculine essence partners each lean into our roles.

THE MASCULINE	THE FEMININE
• Attention, Presence, Action	• Creativity, Emotions, Desire
• Wants to ravish/penetrate	• Wants to be ravished/penetrated
• Dominant	• Submissive
• All about how you relate to the outside world, and the actions you take	• All about how you relate to and reveal your inner feeling states
• Most wants respect from women	• Most wants attention from men

Appreciation of the sacred gifts of polarity are what too many women have traded away in our collective poor bargain. In order to feel safe, secure, and in control at all times, we emulated the men we feared and ended up women in men's clothing, literally. Under the guise of being "strong, independent women," we no longer let ourselves be supported, contained, and held. For the majority of us, expressed polarity is so much more pleasurable, fulfilling, and safe than inverted polarity or a neutralization of sexual energy (which may *seem* safe to our wounded parts).

To start healing from the bait and switch of feminism, we women need to learn how to be contained, both by ourselves and others, so we can more fully enjoy our own feminine essence and all its gifts. And the deliciousness of the masculine gifts of consciousness, presence, and attention are offered to the feminine who, in turn, offers her radiance, heart wisdom, and devotion at the altar of love and erotic union. It turns out that no one is responsible for our safety other than ourselves and God, and we can create the conditions for that safety and align our choices with discernment.

So, what now? How do you rest into your feminine and open yourself up to being ravished by a man who exudes masculine energy?

Well, the good news and the bad news is that *your reclamation starts with you.*

Integrating your inner father and mother, essentially maturing your inner masculine and feminine, will deliver you to a lifescape wherein you can truly choose what kind of woman you want to be.

CHAPTER 3

Mother & Father Woundology

"Stop crying."

"You're fine."

"Don't be upset."

"Go to your room."

"I'm not talking to you until you calm down."

"I'll give you something to cry about!"

Were your tears ever met with any of the above statements growing up? If so, it's likely that you experienced growing up under the care of what Dr. Lindsey Gibson calls "emotionally immature" parents (and she details this phenomenon in her book, *Adult Children of Emotionally Immature Parents*). Let's face it, most of us never got to learn that emotions are alchemical, that crying has an arc, and that feelings come to their own resolution if they're permitted to.

In these familial dynamics, children experience emotional isolation, which is often described as "loneliness in a crowd." These children grow up believing that relationships are lonely places where they feel abandoned and burdened at the same time; they need "alone time" just to find themselves, and they experience emotions, both theirs and others', as problematic.[1]

If you're like me, you grew up believing that your feelings aren't valid unless they have a "good reason" to exist. Therefore, when feelings arise, you scan your lifescape for the *reasons* you're struggling with sadness, disconnection, and desperation.

Additionally, for most of us, the experience of conditional love from our primary caretakers left us with what is referred to by Dr. Alfie Kohn as "contingent self-esteem." Self-worth is fleeting, and it only exists when we secure the approval of others. In his book, *Unconditional Parenting* (required reading for all humans, not just parents), Kohn uses published research to build an irrefutable case for the damaging impact of love withdrawal (think time-outs at best, violence or abandonment at worst) and of rewards and praise as setting up a sense of self that is dependent upon the approval of a parent rather than an inner sense of lovability and adequacy.[2]

We then find ourselves, in our thirties and forties, confronting programs of productivity, success, and unboundaried relationships, growing increasingly aware that they are bankrupt methods of controlling the self-rejection that is festering beneath. We live our lives via a codified belief system concerned primarily with what makes us appear good and right. We use learned strategies to avoid feeling the grief, shame, and fear that we are sure would kill us if felt. We attract repeated patterns of victimhood over and over (and over!) again because the parts of us holding these feelings still demand attention, love, and integration.

Feelings need to be felt. They will keep rattling in the cage until they are finally let out.

Gibson writes, "For emotionally immature people, all interactions boil down to the question of whether they're good people or bad ones, which explains their extreme defensiveness if you try to talk to them about something they did."[3] Emotionally immature individuals have not done the "work" of self-integration or nervous system healing to hold emotional energy in the body (that's all that feelings really are!), and also examine the beliefs that drive struggle (like *if I'm wrong, I'm unlovable*).

Gibson remarks that emotionally immature people are notable for how they:

- "[Overreact] to relatively minor things"

- Are irritated by "individual differences or different points of view"
- Use their child as a confidant
- Are inconsistent: "sometimes wise, sometimes unreasonable" (intermittent reward)
- Focus primarily on their own interests
- Are not self-reflective and do not take personal responsibility
- Are black and white thinkers, not receptive to new ideas
- Are total Debbie Downers, always sucking the life out of the party with negativity, criticism, and paranoia
- Cannot hold space for their own emotions
- Are intellectually objective until triggered
- Experience self-esteem that is contingent upon the compliance of their children[4]

Gibson goes on to describe four general types of emotionally immature parents:

1. Emotional parents: run hot and cold, either helicopter parenting or blatantly neglecting and depending heavily on outside sources for balance. You feel like a therapist in this scenario.
2. Driven parents: nepotistically invested in performance, domineering, and overly focused on results. You feel like a trophy child in this scenario.
3. Passive parents: underdeveloped, detached, and avoidant, sometimes enabling abusive behaviors. You feel forsaken and forgotten in this scenario.
4. Rejecting parents: almost completely detached and not at all present, give the impression that they'd rather be left alone. You feel like a burden in this scenario.[5]

Emotional Maturity 101

Gibson appears to agree with me in that the reframing of self-care, self-intimacy, and self-motivated action lies at the heart of resolving victim dynamics.

According to her, we must first recognize emotional maturity, which she describes as:

- Thinking objectively while remaining emotionally connected to others
- Pursuing what you want without exploiting others
- Having a well-developed life and sense of self based on self-intimacy
- Being honest about your own feelings
- Expressing empathy, impulse control, humor, and emotional intelligence
- Being genuinely interested in other people's inner lives
- Dealing with others directly to solve problems
- Admitting your weaknesses and taking responsibility for your role in conflicts
- Taking initiative to repair interpersonal conflict[6]

I would argue that due to the enculturation that we collectively face, the great majority of us grew up with emotionally immature parents, and, before we start to integrate our core woundology, we will continue to play out the patterns handed down to us. What's important to stress is that despite our parents' greatest efforts, there's really no way they were going to get it right (and if you're a parent, that's true for you—and me—too!). Most childhood experiences are at the hands of two people fumbling around with limited resources to support them as they wade through their own emotional depth.

Unmet Needs & The Good/Bad Split

Since we're wired for survival, we often choose to take responsibility for our wrongness and badness rather than blaming our parents. Even if we were abused, molested, or beaten, it's too fundamentally destabilizing to say, "You know what? My parents were awful. They had no clue what they were doing." Instead, when we feel unloved and unsafe, we internalize the feeling that something is wrong with us and set about curating, lying, performing, and strategizing how to win the approval and affection of our parents. We learn to hide the badness we feel inside, and the "good/bad split" commands our consciousness.

Human mammals experience our fourth trimester outside of the womb, and during this vital time, we literally require love and care. This is not some kind of "nice to have" cute window dressing on top of food and water. When our primary needs are neglected and remain unmet, hungry voids form that we instinctively seek to fill however possible.

The findings from the 1970s "Rat Park" experiment, when Dr. Bruce Alexander sought to assess the chemical nature of addiction, help us to further digest these phenomena. He found that rats isolated in a cage with one water and one morphine dispenser go on to become drug-addicted and eventually kill themselves, but when the rats were relocated to "rat parks," enriched environments with social networks, space, and toys, the rats chose water over morphine. Amazingly, previously-addicted rats would even detox themselves voluntarily when relocated to rat parks.[7] Ripping the foundation from the chemical addiction model (and the notion of the addict as mentally and physically disordered), these elegant experiments tell us that, even in animals, *community* is the prevention and treatment for self-medicating, and that addiction is a relational problem. Many argue that this is one of the reasons that 12-step programs enjoy the persistent success that they do. We're often taught that addiction is a disease, sometimes reduced to a genetic disorder, and all that we can do is avoid the substance itself. The irony is that many so-called addicts are treated with psychiatric drugs, the most habit-forming chemicals available.

I prefer to conceptualize addiction as a symptom of the "I am not loved" mother wound (which we'll explore further) that's fueled by split agendas of different inner protector parts, one of which uses shame in an effort to regulate difficult-to-feel emotions. Most of us simply don't have the capacity to develop intimacy with our feeling states, so we engage all types of distractions to mitigate the pain of being alive and alone with our emotions. For some, it's the pain of emptiness that wants to be filled (boredom drinking). For others, it's the fullness of emotions that are intolerable (stress drinking). Either way, it's our inner experience that we are running from. And often successfully!

It's vital to remember that addictive behaviors are often effective self-management strategies, and that the act of shaming, overcoming, or "trying to get rid of" the addiction itself is grounds for a perpetual cycle of suffering and failure. Instead, one could legitimize the choice and acknowledge the object of the addiction and the associated behavior—*How is this actually working for me?* or *What needs am I meeting by engaging in this behavior?*

When you legitimize the addiction, you create space for there to be a deeper inquiry, such as, *If I were allowed to want something even more than I've allowed myself to want, what would it be?* The resolution and transformation of addictive patterns requires connection to a *Yes* that feels more magnetic than the *No* that the addiction fulfills.

Jean Liedloff explores the roots of our emotional struggles and subsequent addictive pleasure-hunting in her book *The Continuum Concept.* Through her time with the South American tribe, the Yequana, Liedloff discovered ways that North Americans have gone astray. Babies are designed, expectant of, and singularly oriented toward human skin-to-skin contact. In ancestral times and indigenous living, babies are held from the moment they are born until they can crawl (six to eight months), and they are not left out of human contact for one minute. Literally. They are dragged through rain and rivers, bounced around, and exposed to chaotic noises, sensations, and rhythms. Liedloff writes that immediate skin-to-skin contact is so embedded in the evolutionary mother-newborn dyad that in the absence of this imprinting, a mother's physiology begins to prepare for the grief of a stillborn.[8] Our relative distance from our children reveals to us something important about the ever-common "Baby Blues" that mothers have come to expect, doesn't it?

These *co-regulated* Yequana babies are then trusted to make their own decisions around self-preservation. They sit next to large holes in the earth, crawl on the edge of wild rivers, and sample their environment. There is no helicopter vigilance that instills a belief that *they do not have what it takes to survive*. There is no *good baby, bad baby*, no histrionic celebrations when they accomplish something.

Liedloff's manifesto for attachment parenting turns a precious and unrealistic-feeling, holier-than-thou paradigm into a clear and logical mandate: conform to the continuum or cause lifelong suffering. Might it be worth investing six months in your newborn's care if it means that your child will lead life from a core stability?

Because the security of love and touch are basic needs, experiencing a loss or withdrawal of love—or worse—abuse, violence, aggression, or hostility is the existential equivalent of mortal risk. So, for the sake of survival, we learn to selectively curate a persona that is more likely to secure approval. We hide, from both others and ultimately from ourselves, the dimensions of "us-ness" that would seem to threaten connection.

We perform this version of self until we begin to integrate the mother and father wounds so we can reparent our way into sovereign adult living. While there's no codified rubric of mother and father wounds, viewing the woundology through the below lens will help you to explore and ultimately mature your inner dimensions.

The Father Wound

Your relationship to your inner father is the relationship you have to attention, presence, and wise action, both in yourself and others. The father wound can result from emotionally unattuned, absent, or abusive fathers, and it distills into the enculturated belief that *I'm not safe* in these four walls, in this family, and by extension, *I actually don't belong here.*

Core Wound: I am not safe. I do not belong.

Father Wound/ Immature Masculine	MEN	WOMEN
	• Distrust men • Seek female nurturance • Non-initiatory/passive • Peter Pan syndrome • Reactive/defensive • Unreliable • Easily threatened • Can't sit still • Know it all	• Doesn't "need anyone" or ask for help • Feelings need to be fixed or avoided • Vigilant productivity • Impatience • Man criticizing, hating, shaming, controlling • "I'll get him to see"
Integration/ Maturation	• Takes time to respond • Clear boundaries • Clear on commitments • Calm in the storm • Patient • Supportive	• Confident direction • Container creating • Easeful to-do list • Integrity of word • Clear boundaries • Trust in self • Able to sit in stillness • Enjoys challenges

Father-Wounded Men

Father-wounded men come in many varieties, from never-wrong volatile tyrants to the fun-loving "Peter Pan" type. The father-wounded man avoids his own masculine self-actualization and experience of hierarchically surpassing the father he still fears. He rejects his own feelings, and without a mature, actualized inner masculine container, he simply cannot hold his own emotions, tending toward defensiveness, reactivity, and avoidance.

It's pretty easy to spot the father-wounded man. He feels uncomfortable around other men, either semi or subconsciously. He'll seek out female attention and will make fast female "friends." Because he was never truly seen as worthy by his father, he abides in relentless pursuit of external validation. At the same time, he longs for everyone to simply get off his back and otherwise relates to responsibility with overwhelm.

He may feel threatened by the idea of being wrong, which further feeds his desire to become the master of every domain, even if it means prematurely asserting and proclaiming his expertise. It's really tough for him to say, "I don't know." He lacks the capacity to open with curiosity to learn more, and thus would prefer not to know the truth. He's a perfect match for father-wounded women.

Father-Wounded Women

Father-wounded women live in a steadfast energy of *I've got me*, and they prize their capacity to figure it all out without help. This is a woman who's mastered the art of the lone wolf mentality. She resists receiving; it's rare for her to lean into the support of community. Because emotions are often riddled with all kinds of uncomfortable and unwelcome sensations, the father-wounded woman becomes highly efficient at avoiding, distracting from, and blaming whenever difficult feelings arise.

Women who possess father-wounded qualities are often extremely impatient and can reflexively criticize, shame, and micromanage men, thinking that we know better how a man should be a man.

We are the self-identified feminists, the ones who believe (without a shadow of a doubt) that men are fundamentally inferior.

My father wound lives under the neon lights of: "I'll get him to see." In conflict with a man, I'll recruit evidence for my perspective, remaining calm and making my case. Somewhere, I learned that if I suppress my own emotions, hold space for his, and explain, then he'll understand, change, and finally be safe. Other women freeze and go quiet, while others blow up with storms of emotion that they dump on anyone within radius.

When you are arrested in your father woundology, you treat yourself the way a reckless teenage boy would:

- Ignoring your body's signs and cues, pushing yourself with caffeine, touching yourself to take the orgasm, telling yourself to power through
- Yelling at yourself to *get over it* and *stop being such a bitch/diva/baby*
- Reacting with blame and finger pointing
- Lacking a structured but easeful relationship to commitment and follow through

Maturing the Masculine

Father energy can be described as the masculine within us. It's what creates the strong container for the inner feminine, able to resist the poor bargain (unlike the miller in "The Handless Maiden"), allowing you to safely explore your inner and outer environment.

How do you integrate your father wound?

You become an honorable and trustworthy custodian of your body's messages, needs, and desires.

As women, we can set masculine containers for ourselves and actively assess what is needed to support an optimal felt experience, whether that's getting clear on the terms of a contract or making sure you have socks when your feet are chilly. To self-husband means that you create the conditions in your own life for your safety and pleasure because you are paying consistent and devoted attention to what is wanted and not wanted. That means that you must know what you need, know how to say *No* and ask for what's wanted, and never settle for chaotic or insufficient containers. The art of self-fathering or husbanding (because what we long for in a father as a little girl is the same as what we long for in a husband as a woman) renders the inner feminine safe to emerge. This kind of masculine self-containment enables you to remain soft and openhearted but with fierce, clear, and consistent boundaries.

I was called to lean into my own self-husbandry, ironically, through one mundane act of self-betrayal that broke the camel's back. I was meeting my girlfriend to go to a sex shop to buy some new pole dancing outfits, as you do. She was running a bit late, so to appease my inner taskmaster who loves getting things done, I stopped into an unfamiliar car wash service center. As I arrived, I noticed there wasn't anyone officiating the car wash experience—no office or podium or master of ceremonies. The chaotic disorganization of this workflow put me into a bit of a swirl. *Do I stay in the car? Do I get out? Am I meant to pay now, or later? How long does this take? How much does it cost?*

So, I did what I and many women do: I went with the flow rather than establishing clarifying information or honoring the No I felt about the whole experience. I found myself loitering awkwardly on the other end of the washing tunnel, but now, my friend was waiting for me, and I was waiting for a man to hand wipe what felt like every molecule of water off the car, for what felt like approximately seventeen hours.

Now, this gentleman began to ask me friendly questions, including whether I live in Miami and if he could have my Instagram handle. Instead of expressing my need to leave, I wrote down my handle on a piece of paper, fawning in a full-blown stress response. When I finally got into the car, I proceeded to crash it into a pole (very funny, universe) on my way out.

What was my role in this seemingly random string of inconveniences? I neglected to create a safe container for myself by simply "going along" with whatever was happening.

What I could have done was create the conditions for my safety. I could have found someone at the car wash to ask, "How long does this take? How much does it cost? Do I stay in the car, or not?" I could have let the man assisting me know that I needed to leave. I could have said I wasn't available to share my Instagram handle. Ultimately, I could have driven out of the place with a stable, regulated system, and an intact car.

A man who's integrated the father wound is a man who has learned to take time to respond, who's very clear with his boundaries, knows what he can commit to, and who has a very deeply rooted sense of calm in any storm. There's a distinct integrity tied to his word. He is patient, supportive, and directive. He has a capacity for the containment of others, which translates to this juicy, delicious quality for women to be around. He has the capacity to transmit grounding from his nervous system to hers, and he does this quite simply through his presence, his gaze, his touch on her shoulder, or his embrace, with or without contact in his immediate space. The art of self-husbanding calls us to embody these same qualities for ourselves, as we navigate situations on our own.

As you integrate and mature *your* inner masculine (which is an ongoing process and a large part of the work we'll be doing together in Part 2), you'll become adept at creating these conditions for yourself.

When you're ready to become the right man for yourself, it feels like a fierce lion energy grows within. Your spine becomes strong but not rigid, and you access your inner predator, alongside a calm, cool, collected confidence that is never rushed, always attentive, present, and fiercely self-loyal. As you integrate and mature your masculine, your feminine finally has space to flow. So, not only is the inner husband a boundary-keeper and container-setter, but this energy is in service of safety inside and out. Self-husbanded, a woman feels *I've got me*, no matter what, and it's a subtle but important maturation of the help-rejecting *I've got it, I don't need anyone*.

The mature masculine is also extremely adept at holding the overwhelm of uncertainty and confusion. Historically, I would have characterized myself as a pretty competent woman, but in my tenure as a single woman, I have rigorously matured my competencies across multiple realms, including my legal/lawful understanding, management of finances, etc. This past year, I bought a home and leased my first car without the help of a man. Of course, there is the princess part of me that longs for a man to just handle all of this for me. And, yet, to choose to allow a man to handle these dimensions of life, knowing that I could, is an even more powerful form of surrender. This flavor of surrender, offered to a chosen man by a woman who has developed her own inner masculinity, is an opportunity uniquely available to us modern women now.

Developing competencies means showing yourself you've got your back no matter what *and* also knowing when and how to ask for help and support. It's proving to yourself that you can take care of whatever comes your way, even if, and *especially* if you're not the best at it naturally. This is a way of conferring safety to your system while also maturing that inner princess who might imagine somebody is going to come along and save you from all your responsibilities. Your chronic vigilance gets to melt away because you know in your bones that you've got you, and more feelings will be allowed to be revealed and simply felt. A self-husbanded woman is deeply invested in her own impulses, holding space for those impulses to be honored.

43

For instance, one day not so long ago, I had this teeny tiny impulse: *I think I need to cut my hair off!*

It was this tiny *yes*, followed by a big pile of:

Hell no! Are you crazy?! Your hair is your greatest physical attribute and you've grown it through so many painstaking experiences of self-reclamation and it's the longest it's ever been and you'll be ugly and ordinary without it!

Four women at the salon tried to talk me out of it, and I did it anyway. This mundane grooming choice rendered me tearful in the salon chair, not because I was losing my hair, but because I finally felt free to feel the grief of ending my marriage to my children's father over a decade earlier. Was the energy of that experience encoded in the hair that was cut? When we trust our impulses, we play in the mystery of our intuition.

Which brings us to our mothers . . .

Mother Wound

Your relationship to your inner mother is also your relationship to your creativity, emotions, desire, appetites, and sense of satiety. The mother wound reduces down to one simple yet potentially startling phrase: *I am not loved.* It sounds pretty harsh, yet even if it was only true *one time* out of one hundred when you experienced loss or absence of love from your parents, you're bound to have mother woundology. As you integrate your mother wound, this phrase might shift toward compassionate understanding: *My mother couldn't love me. She probably never experienced real love from her parents. She didn't know how.*

44

Core Wound: I am not loved/worthy.

Mother Wound/ Immature Feminine	MEN	WOMEN
	• Fear of being consumed • Afraid of their own feelings/outburst and suppression cycle • Attenuation of inner claim/predator energy • Intolerant of feedback/ emotional rather than vulnerable • Body shame • Wants care and validation from women • Emotional numbness and overwhelm	• Need to earn love, perform • Feel responsible for others' comfort and okayness • Believe connection costs • Attenuation, comparison • Don't know what is wanted or how to ask for it • Attract men who value her structuring rather than her energy • Seek out men who want mothering

(Continued . . .)

Integration/ Maturation	• Attuned to own feelings and body • Create space for feelings • Caretaking impulse • Curious/open • Meet own emotional needs rather than needing partner to change in order to feel okay • Self-soothing, nurtured	• Attuned to what needs to be felt/birthed now • Accept all that is • Feel "something greater is working through me" • Trust desires • Self-care before service • Being over Doing • Receive without giving back • Own what is felt • Accept caretaking • Allow men to fail

Mother-Wounded Men

Mother-wounded men have a crippling fear of being consumed by the "shadow mommy." They grow up to be men who simultaneously resent and appease the women in their lives, experiencing any upset they feel as personal rejection and failure. Often, so-called beta males or "nice guys," these men were compelled to disconnect from their inner predator or masculine aggression from an early age, so their mother could feel okay in the world with her "good little boy." As he grows up, he continues to look to women to tell him what to do and how to do it as rage bubbles beneath the surface of his felt disempowerment.

Let's take a moment to talk about narcissists, shall we? I don't subscribe to the Guild of Psychiatry's ever-expanding bible of what's wrong with humans, since psychiatry does not have a scientifically valid diagnostic system, nor are symptoms ever actually the problem (see my last book, *Own Your Self*, for more on symptoms as sentinels!). However, psychiatry does do pattern recognition well, and there are some behavioral patterns that can be characterized in a manner that will wake women up out of a self-deluding experience of betrayal.

Narcissism is a trauma-adaptation and coping style; narcissistic men experience a profound emptiness inside (described by self-proclaimed narcissists like Dr. Sam Vaknin) and seem to need infinite

45

space.[9] Incapable of true intimacy, they engage lovers, business partners, and friends in parentification dynamics that ultimately result in their continued aloneness. In the "shared fantasy" phase of romantic relationship that Vaknin describes, the narcissist love bombs women to secure the "supply" that affirms and supports an inflated sense of self from his partner. From this woman he needs attention, services, and sex with unconditional support and space.

She, in turn, is both playing his idealized mother *and* also experiencing the longed-for unconditional love of *her* childhood in the limerence or honeymoon phase of the connection. She may enjoy these moments of self-infatuation and celebration and look past the red flags that indicate his lack of fitness as a partner, including intermittent punishment (reactivity, withdrawal of love, or even abuse) that begins to punctuate the love bombing episodes. His mask begins to slip, and once it does, she begins to make demands. He cannot sustain any challenge to his self-constructed identity as a powerful intellect, superlative lover, or rockstar businessman, and so he begins to consciously punish her, intending to destroy the relationship. Only then can he say all the things to her that he wanted to say to his bad mommy, leading her to finally reject him the way he knew she would—and subconsciously needs her to—so that he can finally separate this time through withdrawal of his attention and energy.

In psychology, this behavior is called "projective identification"; the villain within the so-called narcissist is projected without and treated in such a way that the object of the projection begins to act like the villain. In striving to remain the forever victim, he coerces rejection from his woman through his own behavior and then calls her the abuser. Then the cycle begins again in a new relationship with a new woman. While it can be easy to fall into condemnation of such "toxic relationships," these dynamics can be powerful catalysts for self-love and reclamation.

So, what happens when men mature and integrate the mother wound?

They attune better to their own feelings and body. They create space for their feelings and get to experience intimacy with themselves and their intuition. Their souls come to rest in their flesh, and they develop insight into themselves and others. They care and provide from the heart, not through manipulation and strategy. They're curious and open. They know how to offer containment and self-soothe while also holding the capacity for vulnerability with self-possession.

Mother-Wounded Women

Mother-wounded women have a habit of making themselves small because they have been conditioned to believe other women will connect with them more readily this way. They're not only afraid to be wealthy, beautiful, radiant, and audaciously expressed, but they revel in their smallness, constantly self-assessing, critiquing, and comparing themselves to other women. To these women, the act of receiving is terrifying. Receiving a compliment with a simple "thank you" feels like a strenuous task, and receiving a gift is enough to induce a full-blown panic attack. I have felt firsthand how deep this groove runs; how even despite my best intentions, and what I deem to be some pretty hard-earned self-awareness, the mother-wound programming is profound.

I distinctly remember a night when the power went out at my house. Ever the good homesteader, my generator immediately clicked on. So I went outside, looked down the pitch black, dark street, and there my house was: obnoxiously lit up, with my hot pink lights and windows all aglow. My chest gripped. The first thought that I had was: *Somebody's going to come and rob me!* I recognized the absurdity and irrationality of that thought and was able to see the coupling of me-having-more with you-will-be-punished. Having, it turns out, is way harder than you might assume.

The mother wound is where and how we learn to self-betray to secure approval and connection. Though you may mostly conceive of betrayal as a crime committed against you, I promise that if you look at any experience of betrayal that you've had in your life, you were already betraying yourself before that was reflected to you.

Integrated Mother Wound

It may feel dangerous to actualize and integrate the mother wound because it may mean rejection by your mother. On some level, you unconsciously sense that your empowerment may trigger your mother's sadness and the rage she may feel about her unlived life. The inherent compassion you feel for your mother, the desire to please her, and the fear of conflict understandably lead to the habit of self-smalling. This is why one of the most powerful pattern disruptors for mother/sister-wounded women is committing to celebrating yourself with safe women; resolving "commiseration connection" in service of authentic enthusiasm for another woman's expression is one of the ways that we can collectively create that safer world we are truly longing for.

For women, integrating the mother wound is surrendering to the process of life, to God, and becoming a daughter of Mother Earth, herself. Meaning that you align with your body and the natural world, and you tend your divine spark, your child parts, and your whole Self. It is celebrating all that is full, ripe, and wonderful, and knowing that longing never ceases. A mature woman feels and knows in her bones that she's actually here to honor this beautiful vessel with the utmost self-care, prioritizing pleasure, honoring impulses and desire, and anchoring to the truth that just your *beingness* is actually your gift.

As a woman begins to integrate her mother wound, she extinguishes her impulse to apologize for who she is. She fiercely strips away her paralyzing self-consciousness, making way for an expression that is boldly and authentically hers. These women have soft bodies and a relationship to men that is so deeply loving, honoring, and respectful. As she does the courageous work to lean into herself, she can allow her man to fail without feeling like she needs to save him.

Sacred Wound

You may be somewhat familiar with this wound, as it can be easily described as all the "fucked up shit" that's ever happened to you in

48

your childhood that sent you on the path only you can walk. And in that misfit bag 'o horrors, there's often one cardinal wound that whispers one specific sentence over and over and over and over.

The sacred wound influences the lens through which you view your life, and it determines the way you narrate based on what you made that violation, injury, or trauma mean about yourself and the world around you.

This is your story.

The sacred wound can impact and inform your life in two ways; one is that you resort to a "why me?" type mentality, where you believe life is inherently against you. You'll create and look for all kinds of evidence to support the case that your life is exceptionally unfair. The second is where you take all the markers of abuse and adversity you experienced as a child and morph them into driving aspects of your life that you really appreciate on many levels. This is the "life is happening for me" approach, where the sacred wound is seen as something perfectly designed for you to connect with your purpose in this lifetime.

49

When I look at my own life, I can see very clearly how the aspects I appreciate most about myself emerged from and developed from this wound specifically. Like a cosmic joke of sorts, perhaps it's true that there was no other way to get to this version of me without that sacred wound. The self I formed as a result of my deepest woundology exists because it's the one that would help me engage the experience of reconnecting to God across the disconnection and pain. To come home to myself.

When you derive a sense of meaning from that which otherwise seems like random badness and horror, there is a specific kind of delight in the impossible-to-make-up design of it all. I like to say *suffering ends where meaning begins. . . .*

CHAPTER 4

Victim to Vixen

"He who fights with monsters might take care lest he thereby become a monster."

—*Nietzsche*[1]

It's no mistake that your wild, fierce, feminine nature has been hidden from you; this is by design, literally and figuratively.

I've said it many times and I'll say it again, because it's that insidious: the only human pathology is victim consciousness, an illness that is enculturated and entrained into us in our early years of childhood. It's multigenerational, and I would argue that it's socially engineered and reinforced. We inherit stories of all the bad things that happen and marinate in a childhood field of blame, finger-pointing, and zero-sum games.

Victim theories underpin every aspect of our dominant culture:

- **Medicine:** where you're a victim of cholesterol, bad genes, serotonin imbalances, cancer mutations, invisible viruses, biting ticks, and invading parasites.
- **Relationships:** where you're a victim of your toxic ex, your messed-up parents, your unruly kids, or even your trauma.
- **Finances:** where you're a victim of under-privilege and resource scarcity and a debt slave for life.
- **Reality itself:** where we are gaslit against our own senses— common and felt—to believe magical tales including that we

evolved from monkeys, that the wonders of architecture the world over were built in the era of the horse and buggy, that we are on a spinning globe with water stuck to it, and that NASA actors are heroes.

- **Oh, and then there's terrorists, nuclear bombs, and meteor extinctions:** all psyops keeping you arrested in stress physiology.[2]

When it comes to all of the above, life is random, fundamentally malevolent, and you are helpless to do much about it other than worry. Shame and virtue signaling are born from this triangulation against our bodies, nature, and God. Disconnected, we are cut off from our own Source channel, and very readily controllable. Victim conditioning is something we are meant to mature beyond, and it is the root of painful powerlessness and a fragmentation of self that perpetuates a war within, so we are easily baited into wars without.

As my beloved friend Dr. Tom Cowan wrote to me one day:

Underlying these questions is another question which is: How do we know something, as opposed to believing something? There are essentially two ways of knowing something. The first, and best, way is to have a direct, personal experience of that "thing." Then, particularly if the experience/observation is repeated, the experience leaves us with knowledge and certainty about this issue.

The second way of obtaining knowledge instead of belief addresses issues for which a direct experience is either hard or even impossible to come by. In this case, one must use logical, rational thinking and what has come to be known as the "scientific method." . . . [but also] you must then ask yourself, where did this belief system come from, who gains . . . and how does it help me be a free and reclaimed woman by ascribing to this belief?[3]

Beliefs, thoughts, and perception are so important because they inform our physiology. Called "neuroception," the ability to accurately perceive safety and risk is a function that must be reclaimed from our projections and conditioning in order to feel free, sovereign, safe, and empowered. Think of a gorgeous gal walking down an urban alleyway in the dark. She hears footsteps fast approaching, and an entire inner physiological cascade is unleashed: heart racing, quickened breath, sweating profusely, doomsday possibilities dancing in her psyche. But then, she hears her friend's voice coming from the footsteps, the entire cascade reverses, and she might even discharge any remaining energy with laughter. The only thing that changed was her perception. It is imperative for the Reclaimed Woman—really the Reclaimed Human—to command perception and recollect the reality sorter that is the mind.

Without victimhood (and the belief in a random universe of danger and mishap), we cannot be captured, we cannot collude with our own enslavement, and we will never feel small, helpless, or dependent again. We each have the power to render the impossible possible, and it's time to learn how to unlock that gift. The humble origins of victim consciousness begin in our family homes where we learn what is good and bad, right and wrong, permissible and unforgivable.

The Good/Bad Split

One of the most effective forms of trauma-based mind control (and key tenets of victim consciousness) is socially conditioning the good-bad split. Simply put, we are enculturated around "good" and "bad." "Good" behavior is what secures attention, affection, and experiences of love, safety, and security. We are taught to bring forth those qualities to get our needs met. "Bad" is what seems to challenge our connection, since so-called "bad" behaviors make our caregivers unhappy. It's the subtle little things we do (or the not so subtle, "annoying" things we do) that encourage our parents to close their hearts, withdrawing affection and attention for their own self-protection. Where there was once the promise of connection, we receive a cold, icy presence at best, and violence, abuse, and manipulation at worst.

If you grew up in an inconsistent home, unable to anticipate consequences and punishments, your vigilance was refined by the most effective tool that exists in behavioral conditioning. Psychologists call it "intermittent reinforcement," and it's a powerful vector of compliance, obedience, and lasting conditioning.

For women, the good/bad split shows up in neon lights around the Madonna/whore dichotomy. Culturally, the Madonna is the one to be feared or fertilized, whereas the whore exists to be fucked or fetishized, and never the two shall meet. For this particular polarity, denominational religions have played an essential role in the agenda to characterize the body, and notably sex, as dirty, dangerous, shameful, and best kept a secret. Goodness is found outside the body's desires: in service, in piety, and in the realm of devotional thoughts.

The New Age movement of spiritual bypassing hasn't helped the experience of the good/bad divide. Popular exploration of tantra and energetic lovemaking invites white-light, holy "spiritual" sexuality that is reserved for candlelit private chambers, as contrasted by soulless, dirty, grinding, animal sex and flagrant, inappropriate expressions of base sexuality. In this arena, too, we're left feeling that there's good and bad sex, good and bad women, good and bad men. Reminder: whenever we are in that duality, victim consciousness is pulsing right beneath.

It's easy to see the dualistic line of thinking evidenced in the reflexive rhetoric you likely grew up with: *"Be a good girl and behave!"* As we've explored and will continue to, this reflexive rhetoric stems from our parents' own wounding and enculturation; yes, the entrainment is generations deep (which means by doing this work you also have the power to end cycles of pain in your lineage). And the mother and father figures (or whoever is playing those roles) set up the very first victim triangle.

53

Allow Me to Introduce The Triangle from Hell

Take a moment and bring to mind something that is happening in the world right now that's absolutely intolerable to you; it could be an environmental issue, a geopolitical issue, a medical issue, or a health freedom issue. Conjure one of the most extreme examples you can. Now find the sensation in your body that's unbearable to you: the part we might dub "the destroyer of injustice."

Feel this part and connect to her:

What would she scream if she had one line to scream?
What does she want you to do?
What does that part of you need?
What would happen if your inner destroyer of injustice retired?
Who is she protecting?

In this brief visualization, we have met two aspects of Stephen B. Karpman's famous victim triangle (a.k.a. the Karpman Triangle), which he articulated in the realm of conflict resolution and drama/family therapy. This triangular interpersonal dynamic consists of a victim, a villain, and a rescuer.

The victim is the vulnerable one in our visualization, the poor innocent who's attacked, betrayed, forsaken: the one who is in need of protection. And (perhaps surprisingly, if you identify as an activist) your inner destroyer of injustice is actually the villain, an archetype most of us never identify with.

The third member of our agitated cast of characters is the rescuer, another role that's highly familiar to self-identified healers, light workers, and helpers.[4]

The Villain ◢ The Rescuer

The Karpman
Triangle

The Victim

Here's how the roles of the triangle shake out:

VICTIM	VILLAIN	RESCUER
The perpetrated against, the abused, the oppressed, the weak, the powerless.	The perpetrator (who can feel like the savior when in righteousness).	The hero, the savior!
She makes statements like, "poor me, why me, no fair!"	The villain is the bad guy/girl/system at the end of the pointing finger (and also the one pointing the finger).	The victim says to the idealized hero: "Oh my goodness, what would I do without you, my savior, my hero! Thank you so much for showing up and rescuing me!"
She uses phrases like "should, "have to," and "can't" and complaint as a form of connection, and self-soothing.	The external source of power that's "responsible" for your suffering.	The rescuer believes that she's just here to help and assumes the victim is better off for it.
Stress Physiology: Freeze/Fawn	**Stress Physiology:** Fight	**Stress Physiology:** Flight (into action)
Transformational Mantra: "I am radically responsible for my experience."	**Transformational Mantra:** "I don't need anyone to be bad and wrong to choose what's best for me."	**Transformational Mantra:** "I can never know what is best for someone else."

55

This pervasive triangle is predicated on the insistence, by all parties, that *reality should be different than it is*. Powerlessness is the energy that vivifies this shape, a field of consciousness that manufactures suffering, even as it imagines it's blameless or even virtuous. When you're operating from the victim triangle, you can only ever access a surrogate hit of power or self-value.

By definition, victim consciousness is predicated on separation and the possibility that someone is right, and someone is wrong in the face of any challenge. Since victim stories cannot survive without outside energy, victim consciousness is fundamentally vampiric. The greatest irony is that all the characters in the triangle are actually steeped in victim consciousness, dancing with a bad and wrong enemy that they empower. Until you officially exit the triangle, you continue to work through the well-worn grooves of this angular loop, wearing all the damn hats, shuffling around in a Sisyphian-style hell. You will insist that reality be different, you will rest in some degree of superiority or inferiority, and you will experience chronic resentment, bitterness, and disappointment as a result.

We carry our victim stories because, through our childhood patterning, we *were* potentially victimized by someone more powerful who imposed their needs in violation of our own (emotionally, physically, psychologically). As adults, we continue to defer to this mindset and worldview, abdicating the personal responsibility and power of choice that attends adulthood. Over time, living powerlessly does a number on the nervous system.

You've likely heard of stress physiology and know about the different kinds of responses that can be dominant for each of us, whether it's fight, flight, freeze, or fawn. The victim triangle breaks down beautifully into these responses.

When you lead with the victim, you are in your freeze/fawn response, because you feel that there is nothing you can do. The victim holds the belief that we live in a meaningless random universe where bad is bad and good is good. In this "helpless" state, our needs for boundaries and care get met through pity, attention, and coddling. Moreover, our victim stories tend to drive disappointment and resentment, because that is the fetish of the victim.

Maybe your victim story is, as has been mine: "nobody has my back." Maybe it's "everybody always leaves me in the end." "He took advantage of me, betrayed me, and deceived me." "This always happens to me." "I have it harder than everyone else. No one understands me. I'm broke. I'm sick. I'm alone. I'm a failure." "It's in my genes. It's my brain chemistry. I have no luck." The victim requires an outside force to save them, so they throw their hands up and choose complaint over personal responsibility, arrested in powerlessness.

Because our society is so conditioned to seek answers externally, the victim triangle has become an easy trap. This is especially true when it comes to conventional medicine. Why? Because being rescued from your ailments is considered a *safe* way to access a false sense of empowerment. Turns out, when we *identify* with chronic illness, we get something very big out of it. We get to feel comfortably constrained by the limitations of a sick person. We get boundaries. And we don't have to learn to say "no," because if we are sick, we just can't. We get ongoing or immediate care and attention. We get pity and compassion. Most of all, we get to feel right about how messed up and broken we always suspected we were.

Every single woman I ever helped to jailbreak from the psychiatric and medical system came to me believing that something was very wrong with her. In fact, so many of my patients described that the delivery of their first diagnosis felt validating, as if to affirm that felt sense of being damaged: "I *knew* something was wrong with me." It's ADHD. Or major depression. *When what you're experiencing has a name, you can force everyone around you to acknowledge that you've been struggling and suffering.* From there, my patients would take comfort in having a pill bottle with their name on it that they opened every single day. That pill bottle conditioned them to accept as truth an otherwise shameful sense of unworthiness and unlovability.

57

Whereas the victim needs pity, the villain *needs* the punishment and suffering of a declared enemy in order to feel worthy and safer, and thus lives in the fight response. The villain is out to win. But because villains have gone out of style and everyone is now a victim, the villain role can be hard to identify. In the realm of world-saving, I call the villain the "angry activist," which is an energy I am all too familiar with. What's a rung above grief, despair, and terror? It's anger. When you're angry, you have a level of life force that wasn't available in the helpless state. Anger can offer a real surrogate hit of power, yet the resonant energy is the same as that of the victim: *fear.* I dare say that most, if not all, activists are running from very huge fears and deep hurts. I'm talking mega father wounds. The stress physiology of the villain is fight, and thus, fighters derive regulation from fighting the enemy they are mirroring in honor of the victim they project from within.

Deep in exile are the parts of us that hold immense pain. These reservoirs blend with the parts that are also there to make sure that pain isn't felt. We are typically fighting the childhood battle against that bad mommy or daddy, a battle that can never be won in the present.

Activists *say* they "want a better world," but what I've come to recognize over the last couple of years is that *so many activists (my past self included) take pleasure in the world being as messed up as they proclaim it to be.* They project their own sadism outward, the mirroring takes hold wherein they, as Nietzsche said, often become the monsters they fight. Like the mother who screams at her kids for screaming (hysterically shouting "CALM DOWN!"), you become the mirror reflection of exactly that which you are judging. You become the villain as you tell yourself you are taking action for the good of all. Angry activists enjoy their power to pass the hot potato of fear, inducing big sensations in others as they sound the alarm and rally the troops towards enemy grounds. Without an alarm to sound and an enemy to defeat, however, the angry activist is out of a job—so do they really want a saved world?

RECLAMATION MANTRA: THE VILLAIN
"I no longer require anyone or anything to be bad and wrong in order to exercise my power of choice."

This is about resolving the need to be right about the nefarious forces that be and needing them to be wrong in order for you to exercise your empowered choice.

Instead of leaning into your superiority and righteousness to resolve all the problems of the world, consider the following questions:

Next, we head over to the rescuer angle of the triangle, which is where most helpers and healers and do-gooders live. We just want to do our part to raise consciousness, bring in the better world, and educate the ignorant. The rescuer is also the doting wife who is just trying to help her husband make his decisions and organize his life a bit better, and the clinician whose sense of worth is tied to her patient's compliance. The rescuer is the friend who loans money after a mention of financial struggle, without even being asked. She caretakes the imagined and presumed needs of others, professionally and personally. It's one of the hardest habits of all to break because it is so cloaked in virtue and imagined benevolent intent.

The rescuer lives in flight physiology. Flight might sound like running away, but most of the time, the way that flight represents itself is by fixing . . . because, fundamentally, the rescuer cannot tolerate the feeling of the unfixed. It bears repeating that *even* the rescuer lives in victim consciousness. I love encouraging activists (or those of us who are very identified with helping, fixing, and otherwise showing up to do good in the world) to explore the idea that stepping in to save the day is in fact reifying the powerlessness of whomever it is we're supposed to be helping. For the unaware activists, healers, and helpers of the world, the shadow side of their rescuing ways can lead to a dynamic where they believe that those they help can't help themselves, and they actually need the victims to stay victims . . . or they'd be out of a job!

Over time, the rescuer comes to experience herself as the ultimate victim. All it takes is a breach in appreciation for her service to reveal the covert energetic exchange: "I'll do this for you—but you better do with this offer/information/assistance what *I* want you to do with it!" When this unspoken *after all I do for you* energy is exposed, the martyr is born, and the victim crown is passed, formally, from rescuer to victim.

There is a frank intolerance of suffering that attends this elaborate coping mechanism for the rescuer, one that is predicated on *three foundational beliefs:*

1. Altruism is real.

Altruism suggests that you are doing good for someone else's benefit because you have put your needs aside. The reality is that you can never suspend your needs without either subtly or overtly meeting them through some form of strategy or manipulation. Altruism could be considered an indirect form of need-meeting, wherein you meet your need to feel safe as a good and worthy person while leveraging a covert expectation that your act of kindness will be appreciated or reciprocated in some way. Sometimes our deeper intentions live in the shadow realms of awareness, and, when suggested, feel shameful. I'd like to normalize the fact that a sense of significance, value, and goodness all arise from "doing for others" and "saving the world," and when you consciously align with that intention—to feel good for yourself—you might find that your choices shift.

I learned about covert exchanges through my private practice. As long as my patients appreciated the blood, sweat, and tears that I put into their care, all was well, but if a patient expressed entitlement to more of my time and attention than I had given (in other words, didn't fully appreciate me), I felt resentful. I decided to establish my fees such that the exchange would no longer include a hidden tariff of appreciation. It helped balance the dynamic and for me to see more clearly the hidden strings baked into the doctor-patient agreement. This contract was not "for" the patient any more than it was for me; the terms were to be mutually beneficial for both parties, and I had to get clear on what I needed in order for the power to be balanced. There was

61

one patient whom I intuited I should treat for free after her medication taper became so challenging that I was in daily communication with her and her partner, and I became so personally invested in her recovery that I knew I was invested for myself even more than for her. Her ultimate recovery after two years of life on the brink induced by the discontinuation of thirty years of Zoloft felt like a gift to me. So, I followed my intuition around how to navigate the dynamics and exchanges, and my outcomes became more and more predictable.

Then, one day, I asked myself *why* I was practicing any longer, because my focus had shifted from fixing the system to creating a new one I wanted to live in. I learned that it was primarily because my practice offered me a sense of importance. In fact, I couldn't imagine what the world would do without me if I were to stop helping women come off of medication. As I came to source that sense of importance more and more from my Self, I felt less and less compelled by one-on-one work. I also came to see that group-based healing was the zeitgeist of care and that the master-student dyad was fading. Well, it turns out that the world went on as usual when I closed my practice, and I got to experience myself surviving and even thriving through the ending of yet another identity crutch I thought I would be devastated to lose. So, no, doctoring never came from the fact that I'm a good person who wants to help others. I'm not sure it ever really does, and absent the examination of covert intention, there are many aspects of the therapeutic relationship that can serve to disempower exactly whom they purport to want to serve.

2. The victim "needs" you.

The second belief of the rescuer is that the victim needs you to save them. They need you to ride in on your white horse, wave your shiny armor around, and protect them from the wrongdoings of life.

When we help (especially when it is unsolicited), we reify the victim's powerlessness:

- You baby your husband by assuming you need to solve his problems.
- You disempower your children when you do that science project for them.
- You assume your unemployed friend can't access her own creativity when you give her money she didn't ask for.

In these ways and more, your intolerance for another's suffering leads you to declare: "You can't figure this out without me."

3. It's for your own good.
The final rescuer belief belies a sense of superiority. When you believe you know better what anyone else needs, including your own children, you are walking the dangerous line of projection. You are only you. You are not and cannot know what another's experience is. When you act from this place, you are attached to compliance and obedience on the part of whomever you are helping, and we meet, again, that covert exchange. When you truly listen to another without the agenda that says, "I see and know better what's best for you," you create the conditions for their own sovereign self-discovery.

63

RECLAMATION MANTRA: THE RESCUER
"I trust that everyone's journey here is sacred."

The power derived from this mantra comes through the recognition that there is *nothing* that needs to be fixed. Everyone has their own journey, and their experience, needs, and lessons are fundamentally unknowable to you.

Let others learn from life. Let them tap into the creative soil of desperation and even hopelessness. Let their phoenix rise from the ash of adversity. And while you do that, you can listen, offer your open heart, and steady presence.

> *Before offering help, ask, what if I just listened instead?*
> *Before offering my perspective, what if I secured consent by saying, "I'd love to share what I think about this, are you open?"*
> *Before saving the world and others, what if I worked toward authenticity in my personal life?*

So, where is the exit door from the victim triangle?

Embodiment as Activism

The term "embodiment" has so many different interpretations, and I like to think of it as a combination of sensation and awareness. Old me would have met that with an eye-roll. *Of course, I'm aware I'm in this body. And I'm feeling things. That must mean I'm embodied and there's nothing to see here.*

However, old me didn't know what masculine self-containment looked like. She hadn't begun to integrate her father wound, and she didn't know how to hold herself with care. From my vantage point of greater ensoulment, I would argue that the number one credential—as an activist, a light-worker, or a change-maker—is how embodied and regulated you are. That is the greatest contribution to the ripple effect of empowerment that you can offer. Otherwise stated, the most essential form of activism is *getting back into your calm body*.

If the victim triangle keeps us stuck in stress physiology (disconnected from our sense of okayness and from love in all her forms), the goal is to reclaim neuroception and to see with sober eyes. Because of our particular conditioning, traumas, and wounding, we often see and project danger where it doesn't actually exist. There might be a pile of laundry on a chair in your bedroom, and in the dim light of dawn, that laundry looks like an intruder, and your system responds with an intense physiologic response. You make all sorts of decisions

64

based on that assumption. But if your neuroception is reclaimed, if your capacity to regulate and be with yourself is intact, then you will see that it's a pile of laundry, and you will remain self-possessed. We'll be diving into this concept deeply as you explore your *No* in Parts 2 of this book, but let's make sure that you can't ever un-see victim consciousness at work in your life.

8 SIGNS YOU'RE IN VICTIM CONSCIOUSNESS

1. Have To's and Can'ts
Our words are spells; there is so much power in them. So when you find yourself using phrases like "I have to" or "I had no choice," or the most epically cringe-worthy of them all: "I *should* do _____?" recognize how this tricky form of victimhood keeps you trapped inside the belief that you're being held captive by a malevolent universe, when in reality, you don't *have* to do anything. Look at the areas of your life where you may *feel* like you have no choice and shift your language around how you navigate those instances. Swap "have to" out for a more empowering "choose to" or "want to" and see how that shifts your energy, what you have to say, and your intention as you move through the world.

2. Eggs from the Hardware Store
When you insist that someone or something serves you, loves you, or otherwise meets you in a way that they have clearly shown you they can't, you're trying to buy eggs from the hardware store. Which means you're desperately trying to source something from a place where it's just not available, thus setting yourself up for complete misery and suffering. This insistence that you can convert and coerce a situation to meet your needs is a victim trap, and it creates a petulant energy of "you owe me," "how dare you," and "give this to me." It's a cycle born from the unmet needs we experienced in childhood, a

compensation for the experience of wanting something so deeply, knowing it's not available, and continuing to attempt to source it there.

When you begin to recognize that you're trying to buy eggs from the hardware store, you find a tremendous amount of agency and freedom. What you want is not on offer there, it's as simple as that. It's nothing more than an incompatibility of needs.

3. Needing to Fix

Often a sign of the immature masculine, the sense of needing to fix actually springs from an incapacity to allow things to not be the way you want them to be. This could harken back to a time when you were young and your sense of agency was challenged or overridden, and you couldn't leave or make changes that would bring you back to a sense of safety and okayness. Now, as an adult, your okayness depends on you being able to exert your agency by "fixing." Instead of trying to reorder and micromanage what you deem wrong on the outside, try looking inside to remind yourself that you have much more agency as an adult, and you have many more choices than you did as a child, including the choice to let others be their own version of wrong—without you stepping in to "fix" it.

4. Savior to the Rescue

Believe it or not, it's nobody's role to save the world and everyone in it. An extension of the fixing issue, saviorism is a way for a person to assert their will upon the reality around them, even though they can't possibly know what's right for someone else. Most of us don't even know what's best for ourselves, let alone understand the nuances of the needs of others. So instead of assuming you're the best solution to every problem (and that others couldn't possibly be capable of doing hard things without you), consider that every time you present a solution to an unasked problem, you are, in fact, robbing others of their own agency and the opportunity to source their own power and abilities. Focus on you: clean up your own life, evolve your own relationships, and develop a deeper intimacy with *yourself*.

5. The Currency of Complaint

When you engage in commiseration, you're essentially complaining in efforts to connect to others through your strife, your "poor me" stories, your tales of woe. Who doesn't love to complain about their body? Or the trials of your relationship, or your work grievances? It's a tradition passed down through family lines who find comfort in discomfort. But when your interactions with family and friends are predicated on complaint, you're sourcing energy from victim triangle dynamics rather than sharing it from within. Allowing your problems to become the focus of your attention keeps them front and center. Offer your sacred attention to what's wonderful rather than what's wrong.

6. An Inflated Sense of Superiority

In the New Age world of spirituality, it's easy to get caught up in meritocracy. Awakening to new ideas and new understandings can lead you to look around at the "less evolved" and believe that you are now enlightened and therefore better than everyone else who hasn't traveled your road or experienced your lessons. Perhaps you weren't the best person before, but now you're in the hallowed halls of the "awakened."

This linear perspective that suggests you are better now than you were and better than someone who is like you were (or worse) is energetically expensive to maintain. The good/bad split of bad then, good now requires curation of your dimensions, and it also requires that others acknowledge your hard work, making change more dangerous. What if it's just a journey, all of it weird and wonderful, with no one winning more than anyone else, no new you against old you?

7. The Covert Exchange

Disappointment and resentment are the emotional signatures of victim consciousness, often paraphrased as "what the fuck" when expectations aren't met, and the resulting letdown feels personal and targeted. Indignant disappointment can actually be something you *enjoy* in a sick sort of way, as the first blush of disappointment and resentment can sometimes feel arousing. Until that enjoyment is recognized and owned, you can play a very active role in cultivating and co-creating the conditions that create disappointment and resentment. Hence, the covert exchange: you set yourself up through unclear, poorly communicated expectations, inevitably get let down, and then you get to ride the high of righteous indignation.

Be careful when you offer kindness to others that you are secretly hoping will garner you appreciation and gratitude. If you don't communicate what you want from an exchange, you just might be setting yourself up for a feel-good pity party for one. Focus on how you can be real about what you want and need from an experience so you can break the ingrained habit of sourcing fulfillment through the subconscious, co-creative conditions that are going to lead to disappointing energies.

8. Scarcity & Entitlement

Either you feel like there's not enough, and other people get it while you're unfairly left without, or you feel like you earned it fair and square, and the fact that you don't get to have it is bullshit. Growing up, most of us were conditioned around limited resources: money, food, love, attention, water, energy, and more. We also experienced our parents taking from us (without consent) what suited them (called punishment). We experienced comparison to siblings and competition. When behavior was incentivized

> through the coupling of unrelated things (clean your room and you get ice cream), we disconnected from intrinsic motivation and self-sourcing. If, when I get something, there's less of it for someone else, then I better strategize about how to get more. These are the origins of a rupture of trust in self that reverberates throughout a lifetime.

Meet Your Superpower: Choice

It should never feel okay to rest in the illusion of victimhood, and I believe it's designed to hurt. Therefore, this suffering and struggle are ultimately an invitation to transmute and transform, to walk down the non-habitual path, leading with your non-dominant foot. Disrupting patterns allows you to respond with sober eyes to the sight of what is actually in front of you, acknowledge that it's not what you want it to be, and find a more compatible match to your needs; you mature into sovereignty.

Ultimately what jailbreaks you from the victim triangle is a remembrance of choice. Choice is in fact your superpower, but when you don't know you have a choice, you actually don't have one.

For example, I was in literal fetal position, snot running down my face, incapacitated by my fear that my beloved kitty cat Mushu was going to die. He was neutered at a young age, before I adopted him (which I've since learned can, unsurprisingly, contribute to poorly developed urogenital tracts in male cats), and he experienced a series of four unresolving urinary occlusions before he was two years old. I tried every remedy under the sun I could think of or intuit to help him: cold laser, homeopathy, herbs, and prayer, and called on all the support I had. After what felt like an interminable window of mutual suffering, I took him to the vet emergency room.

Mind you, as a sovereign, biohacking, homesteading mother, I have *never* been to an emergency room for myself or my children. I found myself in the parking lot, shook, sobbing with Mushu by

69

my side, when suddenly, from deep within, arose the remembrance. I remembered the consciousness I teach participants in my lifestyle medicine program, Vital Mind Reset. I remembered the dedication and commitment I have to remaining in the seat of my power, no matter what comes up.

This was my internal dialogue:

Kelly, you don't have to do this. You don't "have to" bring Mushu to the emergency room. Things could shift in two hours. Someone could send you a resource that changes everything, he could spontaneously recover on his own . . . you don't have to bring him here.
You have a choice.

So, I took him in and engaged the system from my power of choice. I chose to bring him into that emergency room.

Remembering your power of choice returns the locus of control within. Even if someone is chopping off your hands, like the maiden in the tale, you have a choice about how to narrate what's happening, through radical acceptance around what actually is and an orientation toward the inherent meaning of all that we live into.

The responsibility of choice can feel like a burden until you begin to enjoy and delight in what's on the other side of *literally* every challenge that you experience, without exception. Soon, you'll begin to love feeling in the dark for your choices far more than you loved "having to" tolerate and go along with all that was wrong in your lifescape.

CHAPTER 5

The Erotic Caress of the Enemy

In a *Law of Attraction* universe of resonance and mirrors, a subtle but palpable sado-masochistic dynamic can take hold. The sadist in this dance is the universe herself: a hard-knocks teacher offering lessons and tests "for your own good." That's how I've sometimes related to the unexpected experiences of adversity or betrayal that come my way. I would submit to my "deserved" experience of pain, grief, shame, and fear, and quickly try to extract the meaning.

What's in this for me?
Why is this happening?
How is this actually serving me?
What in my upset am I being invited to love and attend to within?
How is that which I'm judging on the outside showing me disavowed
    parts of myself?

I started to feel myself bracing against the tough ways I might make the acquaintance of my fears and shadow parts. Like: *Okay universe, bring it on, I promise I'll own it and take full responsibility! But also, please be nice to me!*

That's why, when I learned via Carolyn Lovewell's game-changing book, *Existential Kink,* that the play of kink power dynamics could all be occurring *within me,* that I could be both the sadist and the masochist, something in me *laughed with the delight of recognizing an obvious truth.* We pretend that this is all happening *to* us so that we can have the experience of playing hide and seek with our own consciousness. And so, what if, as Lovewell says, "having is evidence of wanting"?[1] What then?

What if everything is already okay . . . more than okay? What if everything is already exactly how we actually want it to be? And what if it actually feels arousing and pleasurable to pretend to fight with what is through lack, blame, complaint, and self-pity?

From this place, the journey feels a lot less like a spiritual boot-camp and a whole lot more like divine play.

For example, I find insects disgusting. My cats sometimes have fleas. I hate that this is happening. But of course, I *know* that nothing is random, that this can't be explained through a mechanical universe because my girlfriends' cats *also* go outside, and they do *not* have fleas.

I have played with the idea that I am energetically making them vulnerable to parasitism because I'm not protecting their energy fields, metabolizing my negative energies sufficiently, or otherwise burdening them. Even though that's interesting and plausible in my spiritual universe, it feels condemning and, in some ways, leaves me helpless. But what if the truth is that I actually enjoy that they have fleas?

Several times a day, I've brushed my cats and flushed the gross writhing vampires down the toilet. My cats love the caresses and attention. They purr, and I feel like a heroine taking care of them, vanquishing the invaders. As sick and gross as it is to consider that I am fulfilled by this reality, if I move through the shamewall and connect to the feeling of "winning against the fleas" in honor of my beloved animals, I liberate this sadistic part of me into my consciousness. I could then find other ways to connect to and protect my animals that don't require blood-sucking insect dynamics!

The Delicious Feeling of Victimhood

Your superpower of choice can often guide desires, but what about *unconscious* desires? Shadow desires that are being fulfilled as we speak, in the aspects of our lives that we "don't like." Ones we might feel ashamed to acknowledge. To frame our struggles as a source of pleasure may feel like a stretch, but if we focus on the feelings, the sensations in the body that come with the chosen experience, we get somewhere interesting.

Let's say that I received an accusatory email from someone. I might feel a rush of energy up my core, and my stomach simultaneously feels like it's dropping out of my body. It turns out that this sequence of sensations is almost indistinguishable from the sensations that arise when I'm on a rollercoaster or watching horror movies (*which I tell myself I enjoy!*) or even making prolonged eye contact with a tall, strong, handsome gentleman. The difference between the sensations of pleasure and pain, fear and excitement, lies in agency, consent, and choice. Which is why being flogged against my will is quite a different thing than being flogged by an adoring lover. So, what if the experience of the victim dynamic with this "accusatory" person is also something I actually want? Why would I want that?!

When I get to feel victimized in a dynamic, I enjoy feeling the deliciousness of righteous anger, which is admittedly one of my personal favorite feelings. I get the compassion of my friends and the exhilarating energy field of groupthink finger-pointing. I get attention. *And* I get to feel innocent, vulnerable, and feminine. And *then*, if I choose to retaliate, even if just in my mind, I get to flip from more masochistic enjoyment to the sadistic enjoyment of feeling my power over another. I get to meet the wicked part of me that delights in her evil queenship of punishing energy, all without even saying a word. The victim field can be blissful. To fail to recognize the pleasure of enacting your usual role in the victim triangle is to hide from your already *fulfilled* desires.

The shamewall that obscures your desires is the threshold of your shadow, hiding all of the polarities you house. If I think of myself as kind, my cruel punisher is in there. If I'm a loser, my all-powerful girlboss is in there. If I'm consciously identified with my love, light, and glitter feminine, my dark feminine destructress is lurking in the dungeon. Basically, when you're really attached to something, latent in your shadow is the desire to experience the opposite. If you really consciously hate something that is happening, it is worth considering that in your shadow is the desire for it to be exactly this way, as is fear of experiencing the opposite of what you hate. Lovewell writes: "In fact, the conscious mind worries about all this 'bad stuff' and thinks about how to avoid it, but that worry is secretly (shadowily) a kind of erotic caress, an obsessive dwelling with rapt fascination on the face of the very beloved failure and humiliation."[2]

As an activist, I've kept many erotically caressed lovers. For the better part of ten years, I was in a deeper relationship with the anonymous victim and a more arousing dynamic with the identified enemy than I'd ever be comfortable acknowledging. There were moments over those years where I became literally obsessed with the chess moves unfolding on the enemy's side of the table, waiting for the next bill to drop stripping us of vaccine exemptions, the next indication that smart cities and social credits were just a false flag away, and the latest page from the rinse-and-repeat virus hoax divide-and-conquer playbook. It turns out that offering my vital force energy to the enemy's game plan and tactics was an effective avoidance strategy for harder truths in my own life. These dynamics are infused with eros, and they feed us, just not in the nourishing kind of way.

So, do we really get off on these struggles?

Eroticized Wounds

I learned this phrase from Robert Augustus Masters, who explained to me the concept of *eroticized wounds* and the ways in which our cardinal traumas and associated beliefs take on the qualities of erotic attraction as we continue to encounter the same patterned dynamics of rejection, betrayal, and abandonment as adults.

If you were sexually abused, dehumanized, or objectified in childhood, you might be confused and disturbed to realize that you are turned on by experiences that induce similar feelings. It's more than just attracting what's familiar. It's *wanting* to experience it and deriving enjoyment and pleasure from fulfilling this desire.

For most of us, when we experience pain and injury (whether emotional or physical), the circumstances and markers of the experience get tagged with a particularly strong charge. More than just a survival-oriented warning system, prevalent psychoemotional patterns would suggest that the very same circumstances and conditions of our early struggles become how we experience love and aliveness as adults. Neglect, gaslighting, abuse, and volatility can all feel like a cozy homecoming arrived at through varied front gates.

Why would we ever do this to ourselves? It's so incredibly counterintuitive, yet as humans, these painful wounds become the bonding points we seek in partnership and beyond. Maybe we do so that we can have the opportunity for completion, an opportunity for our adult selves to stand up for our child selves. Or so we can begin the journey of self-reclamation, revisiting these spaces with a renewed sense of compassion, tenderness, and enlightened awareness, allowing us to embody and choose to experience them. The more this reality can be consciously acknowledged and *approved of,* the more *liberated shame energy* becomes available.

Shame is never easier to hunt than in the realm of erotic fantasy. Shame is the energetically expensive resistance to the seemingly irreconcilable tension of opposites within, one that says I want this, and the other that says you shouldn't. We keep our lifelong fetishes cloaked and hidden, often because they feel inexplicable. In doing so, we neglect one of the most powerful realms of reclamation: the hurt that lies beneath the desire and arousal that itself beckons us home.

For example, in his groundbreaking book *Erotic Mind,* Dr. Jack Morin discusses a woman who was sexually abused in childhood. In her adult life, she goes on to enjoy what she calls the "soulless, loveless, objectified experience of promiscuity and sex." In so doing, she eroticized her childhood wound so as to become the "slut who seduces, rather than the worthless garbage that was violated."[3] By engaging consciously with this kink, she is granted a ripe opportunity to rewrite her narrative into one where she can reclaim her vulnerability and intimacy as *power*, rather than playing out the same wound to protect herself from the pain of her former abuse. Childhood discipline and punishment fears also fuel adult fantasies and what Morin dubs our "core erotic themes," explaining that we often delight in the triumphant power of choosing to engage what was once imposed upon us. He reminds us that excitement lies in attraction and that sexual energy and arousal thrive in the realm of the taboo.

When you can engage with these imprints in intentional ways, you free up space to peel off the husk that is the pain body, leaving you with a beautiful, powerful playground experience of power, desirability, worthiness, and pleasure—perhaps *even* with some of the flavors of the pain of your childhood, but now through your own conscious choice.

When you acquaint yourself with your disavowed desires and consciously feel the previously unconscious pleasure and fulfillment in scarcity, being controlled, wronged, humiliated, rejected, or offended, life becomes a play, a game, and you get to reclaim vast energetic resources. Lovewell says that we "become lucid in the dream of waking life, capable of executing marvels. We become undeniably, tangibly aware of the divine presence, the spark of Godself within us."[4]

So, let's play . . .

CHAPTER 6

Self-Initiation

Only a fool is interested in other people's guilt, since he can-
not alter it. The wise man learns only from his own guilt.
He will ask himself: Who am I that all this should happen
to me? To find the answer to this fateful question, he will
look into his own heart.

—Carl Jung[1]

The Path Home to Yourself

Spoiler alert: The self-initiation journey is not an easy path, but neither is a lifetime arrested in victimhood. Initiation requires rupture, and it is existentially terrifying, by design, but an expanded experience of okayness awaits.

As mentioned, the tariff paid at the portal to any expansion seems to involve the loss of something we thought we could never live without: a loved one, a marriage, a job, an identity. The handless maiden loses her hands (her connection to nourishment, pleasure, others), and with that much less to lose, ventures forth in a way she wouldn't have if not for that devastation. In her seminal book, *Guiding Principles for Life Beyond Victim Consciousness,* Lynne Forrest illuminates that the payoffs for staying stuck and small can include: "a sense of belonging, a sense of accomplishment, career advancement, emotional safety," and I would add: a sense of being good and right.[2] This makes up much of the poor bargain: a false concept of masculine containment.

But one day there will be a breaking point where the patterns you've inherited from your family and sociocultural programs get more and more intense, such that the experience of your old way of being is so intolerable that you summon the courage to walk into the wild unknown. Through your heroine's journey, you are granted access to the energy that would otherwise be holding the good/bad split intact, so you get to feel more "free" and have a broader range of flavors of self to draw on. You get more resiliency, less vigilance, less fear, and more of the ineffable sense that we are living the life we came here to live rather than surviving to die!

That is the work that we are doing here together. This is your self-initiation. So get excited! Because as women, we *came* here to alchemize, to create, to work through the magic that our bodies are designed for. Now, before we set out into the forest and get real about your big *No*, let's expand the permission field.

Permission Field

You know what a permission slip is: the power to do something, conferred by someone else. We are relational beings who give each other permission through non-judgment, space holding, and approving witness, and it only takes one other person to give yourself the permission you're ready to claim. I know because this is primarily what I did in clinical practice for a decade with women so "mentally ill" they had been told there was little to no hope of them being anything beyond a good patient and taking their meds forever. I gave them permission to no longer see themselves as broken. I offered a reframe, and that transmission shifted the scenery so that they were suddenly the main character in an entirely new play. Now I'm here to do the same for you. A permission slip is useless, however, if you're not going to actually do the thing.

Consider this your permission slip to:

No longer believe you're broken.
Do things differently.

Be the villain in the privacy of your own mind.

Love money.

Stop trying to save the world.

Own your well-intentioned shitty behavior.

Admit when you're enjoying playing small.

Love pity, attention, and being right about how wronged
you've been.

Be audacious and unapologetic.

Celebrate every damn thing about who you are.

Get it wrong.

Get it right.

Release the concept of right and wrong.

With all your dimensions, parts, and fragments invited, it's time to
self-initiate into the full expression of you-ness so you can finally live
and create from the fierce feminine fire you were born to embody.

79

PART 2

NO

CHAPTER 7
The Underworld

Free from all old stories I've been told, I walk through the
valley of my own shadow.

—Yaima, *"Gajumaru"*

The Forest

With stumps where her hands had been, the Handless Maiden still managed to flip a ladylike bird to the life she had known, and she retreated to the forest. Walking for hours, her eyes slowly adjusted to her new life, as did her gait; the soles of her feet became bloodied, bruised, and eventually caked with healing mud. After her first night of wandering, she had a new glint in her eye, an opalescent gleam that spoke of other worlds and things that you and I have never seen. She became a woman of the forest, a nymph with earth in her steps and twigs braided into her hair, without hands or a name.

The Handless Maiden walked through the seemingly endless woods. Wind whipped through her, stripping away her old self and showing her the pillars of strength and power that had been inside her all along. But as the hours stretched long, hunger settled heavily beneath her heart. Without food, she would soon starve . . .

She started to grow so weak with hunger that she cried out prayerfully—to God, to Source, to something Greater—for help. And because there is always mercy available when a maiden cries out for help from her tender, vulnerable (if bruised) open heart, the heavy shadows of the forest lifted, and a lush vista revealed itself in the distance, not too far away. She was, in fact, at the edge of the royal orchard that was replete with pristine rows of pear trees, perfectly ripe for the plucking. Unfortunately, a wide moat stood between her and sustenance, and she was all but bereft with no way to cross, so close and yet so far from nourishment all at once.

Just then, an angel-like spirit adorned in long, white, ethereal garments and radiating an internal luminosity that glowed like crushed pearls heard her prayer and materialized before her. As the maiden walked toward the orchard, the serene, peace-inducing figure drained the moat, as if seas parted for her. Once across, the maiden's eyes drank in the immaculately attended rows of pear trees with the spirit by her side. Each pear was perfectly formed, and every tree perfectly balanced, with no pear out of place, and no branch left unadorned.

It was a sight to behold! By the light of the moon, she tilted her head back to bite a pear from the tree, the stumps of her wrists gently holding the fruit in place as she pierced the skin, juice running down her chin. It was the most ecstatic meal of her life, lit by soft moonlight.

She was spotted by a gardener, who almost couldn't believe his eyes. An angel and a woman without hands; *this must indeed be magic!*

The next day, when the king (he was young, fresh-faced, and Hallmark-handsome) came to gaze upon his beloved pear trees, he noticed right away that the moat was dry and one of his carefully cultivated trees was missing a perfect pear. The gardener told him of the mysterious woman and her holy companion. Intrigued, the king asked the gardener and his magician to join him that night to see if they could spy the same scene. He was sure that his magician would know of these matters.

And so, by moonlight, the king, the gardener, and the magician held watch until their eyes trained upon . . . her.

The maiden of the forest, as much dirt as woman, accompanied by the glowing white spirit. As she approached one of the pear trees, the limbs bent towards her, offering a benediction of its life-giving fruit. She sucked and ate without hands, pear juice raining down over her form, leaving clean channels through the mud that caked her face and neck, and the young king fell in love, wordlessly. He approached with wonder and respect.

"Who are you?" He asked.

"Who am I?" she repeated, and something stirred in the young man. He could see she was in this world but not of it.

"Is she a woman or a spirit?" He asked the magician.

"Both." The magician replied, recognizing the living miracle before him.

The king knew that, regardless of her social status, her wild woodland appearance, and the fact she'd helped herself to his prize pears, she was meant to be his bride. Right there, in front of his gardener, his magician, and the silent angel, he bent to one knee and offered her his whole heart, and she accepted.

She left the woods to live with him in the castle, and made her home with him, their lives entwined. He loved her with great tenderness, and even had his most clever silversmiths craft her a pair of silver hands to bring her ease, yet she hardly wore them, preferring gentle gauze. The king's mother lived with them, and she adored the young queen as well. The admiration, respect, and expansion were mutual.

One day, the king was called off to war in a distant kingdom. Bidding his mother to message him if his bride grew full and round with the fruits of his love, he left to defend his lands.

Within months, it became clear that the maiden was with child. She took delight in her growing body, felt at home in herself in a fresh new way, fell more in love with the life inside of her each day, and met dimensions of herself that had only whispered to her in her former life.

She gave birth to a healthy, vital boy, with all ten fingers on his perfect little hands: the kingdom's new heir! The old queen sent a dispatch to the king to inform him of the joyful news.

The messenger who was tasked to deliver the message made his way to the king with pride in his stride and made a good pace until the woods became very, very hypnotic. After a while, he could barely keep his eyes open. He fell into a deep slumber by a stream. Recognizing an opportunity, the devil approached, and traded his note for another:

The young woman gave birth to a half-human, half-dog.

Shocked, the king couldn't believe the tragedy in those words. Yet after he regained his composure, he penned a reply:

I love and accept my wife and my son.

The messenger made his way back to the castle, yet once again he fell into a slumber, and once again the devil switched the missive to make dark mischief.

They cannot live. Cut out their tongues and eyes so I know that it is done.

The queen sobered at this note. She could not believe the cruelty of her son, and she felt burdened with shame and shock. She had come to love the young woman and could not bear for any harm to come to her beautiful newborn grandson. So, she secretly asked a page to sacrifice a deer, saving the eyes and tongue as proof of their death.

The queen then implored the maiden to leave the castle; the maiden resisted flight, for she had no interest in returning to the forest. "Not again," she told the queen, the woman who treated her like a daughter, even though she had come to them a wild woman of the woods, without hands.

"You must flee! You and the babe must find safety in the woods."

And so, she helped the maiden hide the babe under layers of soft fabric and a generously warm cape. The handless maiden returned to the forest, her baby nestled into her breast, throwing herself, once again, into the now familiar yet ever strange wood, and the surprising acts of kindness she trusted would be forthcoming.

To be continued . . .

THE RECLAIMED WOMAN

No

Welcome to your *No*: the forested underworld of dark feminine alchemy, where your problems are your power, and your gifts lie on the other side of your fear.

Empowerment isn't what we've been told it is. It's not taking back what was stolen and winning; it's about owning what you've always had and ending the war inside.

Reclaiming your *No* is about developing awareness and intimacy with the *No* on the outside of you, where you end and the rest of the world begins, and also the *No* on the inside of you, or where you are rejecting, hiding, and then projecting vital parts of yourself. *No* is about setting strong boundaries, making clear decisions, taking wise action, and holding bold space for whatever arises, moves, or shrieks in the night. *No* is the pattern disruption that creates the opportunity for meaningful change.

Empowerment requires that you defy the reflex that it will "cost too much" to leap away from your old defensive patterns, stare into the wanting face of what you've been avoiding, and choose uncertainty. It requires that you grow the capacity to feel the shame that gatekeeps your heroic leap. This shift defies the illusion that walking in the well-worn grooves of your *poor-me, no-fair, I-hate-this* story is good enough for your experience as a woman. Your sovereignty asks for an initiation beyond your worst and deepest fears so you can finally reclaim your human superpower: *choice.*

When the maiden steps over the liminal threshold into the forest, leaving her mother and father behind to reparent herself, spurning the luxurious life that no longer fits her, and to realize a deeper kind of attunement, she reaches a major rite of passage in her maturational journey. She accepts her vision quest and the conditions of her self-initiation, much like you, dear reader, since you have made it thus far into the woods of Part 2 and finding your *No.*

As the Handless Maiden gets used to the forest, she becomes familiar with the recesses of her psyche. She rewilds herself and makes contact with her dark witch, Kali, Medusa, bad bitch energy that destroys in the name of love: identities, habits, stories, and too-small boxes of womanhood. The awakening of this darker energy, the cauldron of smoldering eros that lies beyond our appeasement, compliance, and obedience, requires that you move through conditions that you imagine would annihilate you. Yet, you'll find in these transitions the sweet annihilation of becoming, when all that seemed static and fixed pixelates into sparkles of numinosity and recollects anew.

Our maiden, a newfound creature of the forest, taps into her deeper hunger, which Estés reminds us is a woman's desire for true nourishment. The feminine figure in white leads her to food, a guiding light as she enters the underworld of the unknown.

Regarding the pear tree, Estés illuminates:

> *Eating the pear nourishes the maiden, but a more poignant action is this: the unconscious, the fruit of it, bends to feed her. In this sense, the unconscious bestows a kiss of itself upon her lips. It gives her a taste of the Self, the breath and the substance of her own wild God, a wild communion . . . The remarkable idiom of the story is that during the darkest times in the feminine unconscious, Nature feeds a woman's soul . . . It quells the hunger so we can go on . . . toward our knowing destiny."*[1]

You'll notice that even amidst her *No*, the maiden discovers delightful *Yes's*. She has given up her old life and lost her innocence in favor of a life more fully lived. The caresses of nature, of self-love, and the reunion with her own inner nature provide soul-level nourishment and redirect her consciousness toward her true Self. The *Yes's* along the path enable her to keep going, much like the spirit in white who assures her that she is on the right track, the true path home to Self.

Masculine Self-Containment

Here's the plot twist: You're feeling the call to *woman* with more wildness, authenticity, enthusiasm, creativity, and pleasure, but what if you don't need help cultivating those feminine qualities? What if the first and most essential step on the path home to your feminine nature is actually *conferring safety to your system?*

In many ways, my first book, *A Mind of Your Own*, was about conferring safety to your body, and my second book, *Own Your Self*, was about conferring safety to your mind. In this section, you'll learn what it takes to confer safety to your beautiful heart.

You might remember that father-wounded women are set up to embark upon the journey of delivering to themselves the masculine experience of safety that could have come from their fathers but did not. When it comes to self-initiation, however, the compensatory, "I don't need anyone," strategy won't do, and you are called to mature this defense into a deeply resourced, "I'm here for me, unconditionally." Perhaps then, and only then, can your true divine nature unfurl.

The *No* phase is the initiation of your inner father, king, masculine energy into sacred guardianship of your precious feminine *Yes*. When I refer to an inner masculine, it is, in most ways, a rhetorical strategy to allow for the identification of certain inner signatures that result in particular thought forms and behaviors. If you look at the young king, who loves our handless maiden wholeheartedly, as an aspect of the woman's psyche, he represents awakening to self-awareness and masculine self-containment. In fact, the prince/king in every fairy tale can be seen as the arrival of the devotional animus/inner masculine that is finally ready to kiss her alive and escort her beyond princesshood and into maturity. According to Estés, when the maiden is seen by the magician, the gardener, and the king, she is visited by "three mature personifications of the archetypal masculine. They correspond to the sacred trinity of the feminine personified by the maiden, mother, and crone."[2] This part of the tale in the heroine's journey is likened to assembling your team or meeting your

89

inner mentors in the Campbellian hero's journey arc: finding the aspects of your psyche that represent your inner resources available 24/7, at your service.

In the king, the maiden meets a man who can hold space for her, who will do anything for her, who can love her not in spite of but *because* of her wildness. In the words of Estés: "He recognizes her as his own, *not* in spite of her handless, wildish, wandering state, but because of it. The theme of being so without, and yet so sustained, continues. Even though we wander about in an unwashed, forlorn, semi-blinded, and handless state, a great force from the Self can love us, and holds us to its heart."[3]

An expressed polarity is established, and complementarity emerges. By inviting that masculine king in and seeing his strength as a gentle, loving container where your queen can freely play, you heal your own father wound and become the strong masculine presence you need, without violating, entrapping, armoring, or abandoning the strengths available to your feminine essence. You now have more of what it takes to lean into what was formerly avoided because you know the gems are in those caves. And that is who you will become for yourself in this catalytic part of your journey, woman.

In Part 1, we unpacked the father wound, the place where your unmet needs led you to believe you were fundamentally unsafe. Instead of believing that your parents struggled with their own emotional immaturity, you came to believe that YOU are the root cause of your emotional abandonment. The relationship with your inner father is your relationship to attention, presence, and wise action. If you feel like you're somehow lacking in these areas, you'll often put on a show for others, so they don't see (and you don't see) the parts of you holding painful fears and self-doubt. Because the father-wounded woman only knows how to avoid, quick-fix, and judge her inner feelings, she sees her emotions as an annoying problem that needs to be fixed instead of as an alchemical invitation to growth and transformation, a navigational guide on her reality trip.

Self-husbanding isn't about becoming the man you need in your life. Instead, it's about learning what you want and asking for it while standing in fierce alignment with yourself, assessing, discerning, and creating the conditions for those needs, preferences, and desires to be honored. I like to say that it starts with acting like you actually give a shit about yourself. Your inner masculine is always on the job, attuned, and attentive, never whoring you out into not-quite-right, it's-fine, suck-it-up-and-stop-complaining situations.

With self-awareness comes personal responsibility, and your inner husband is ready to take it on. As Jungian analyst Marion Woodman says, "discipline . . . means seeing yourself through the eyes of the teacher who loves you. We have that teacher within ourselves."[4]

Self-husbandry looks like:

I am here for me, in devotion.

It is the art of maturing a strong masculine container for yourself so that you can feel well-resourced, no matter what comes up. As a self-husbanded woman, you know that you've got you, because a dimension of your energy is tasked with assessing your inner and outer safety, and now, the right dimension of you is on duty: your animus Self with a capital S, rather than your protectors hoping to connive, coerce, manipulate, lie, steal, and cheat just to survive.

We are, collectively, in the midst of an epochal paradigm shift, from an era where safety is achieved through external variables to one where it is accessed internally through full self-possession and self-trust. I like to envision this embodied state as a strong spine, soft heart. When we navigate the world this way, we don't give anything we don't want to give, and we always show up as who we are. A good inner husband creates the conditions to hold fear and shame so that a little *Yes* can be born despite inner resistance and a little *No* can be honored despite go-on-just-push-through-it programming. The unspoken script quiets, and the *fuck why did I do that* reflex extinguishes, as does chronic resentment, complaints, bitterness, and the victim stories, because now responsibility, choice, clarity, and discernment oversee the aliveness that animates every moment.

That's not to say that when you adult in this way, you'll no longer get tested or triggered. The devil may still change the messages you get from others, triggering your inner child parts to assume they're being disowned. I believe that our triggers and defensive habits are lifelong companions, but that you will have the space, slowness, and awareness to guide yourself through the alchemy available in every upset.

From this point forward, everything—and I mean everything—that tests and triggers you is an occasion for alchemy.

Feel It, Face It, Free It

When it comes to feminine reclamation, I love to follow the "Feel it, Face it, Free it" order of operations. "Feel it" is all about fully feeling your unwanted, inconvenient, and uncomfortable feels so you can alchemize those sensations in your body through somatic experience. That is where your *No* journey starts and where you come face-to-face with your victim story, the storyline tasked with avoidance of these deeper emotions. "Face it" asks that you explore the mirror, the projections, and how you can see yourself in the perpetrator, find meaning in the stuckness, and then choose what's in front of you. Also known as shadow work, you relate to judgment as a chaperone, introducing hidden parts of yourself to your own awareness. With your upset as a portal, you'll be able to recognize why you don't have what you think you want (hint: it might actually be because a substantial part of you doesn't really want it) and transform old fetishes for struggle and suffering. "Free it" is making art out of your shit and expanding your capacity to have and hold what you say you want.

Consider this body of *No* practices to be your invitation to step away from avoidance and into choice so that you can courageously move in the direction of embracing a different story, a narrative that does not require anyone to be wrong and does not lead to blame or finger-pointing. Unobstructed by your shamewall, your channel of vital force energy will be restored, and you will begin to experience yourself as a conduit for expansion, joy, and peace. Because your relationship to desire will be mature, healthy, and founded on deep trust, you'll start truly manifesting, achieving, and securing *exactly* what you want.

Spoiler alert: If every aspect of the tale represents a part of the woman's psyche, then even the predator lives within you! And when the devil mixes the messages, Estés so poignantly writes, "These are the means by which the predator changes the life-giving messages between soul and spirit into death-dealing messages that cut our hearts, cause shame, and even more importantly inhibit us from taking rightful action."[5]

Together, we will wade into alchemical tools and tactics that can and will heal the great divide inside, the fear-based war between your inner masculine and feminine, and the various parts representing those dimensions, so you are able to embrace all aspects of you.

"No" Disclaimer:

This is not a spiritual meritocracy, and it's not about bettering yourself so that you can finally be lovable and worthy of goodness in life. In fact, in the later stages of masculine maturation, part of the ongoing work of *No* is neutralizing rejection, including the rejection of the former versions of yourself, your mother, and your motherline. We are not going to take that poisoned bait. You're about to discover that you don't have to be a "good" person, and that, in fact, we are all "mixed objects" made of good and bad, responding from old programs until we liberate ourselves to fully choose life and to experience the present moment.

Welcome to your *No*, woman.

RECLAMATION REMEDY: THE ART OF SELF-HUSBANDRY

To light your forested path, here are a few ways to practice the art of self-husbandry and offer yourself some exquisite masculine self-containment.

First things first, grow your capacity

I believe in a hierarchy of needs; first, we must send a signal of safety to the nervous system so that we can explore hidden feelings, unlock caverns of parts, and begin to engage identity plasticity and shifts that would otherwise threaten annihilation. Emotions are *energy* in the body, and, in order to stay centered while that energy is moving, we must grow our capacity to *feel*. We must learn *how* to feel feelings and practice staying open and approving of them. This is why I remain a strong advocate for my 44-day health reclamation program Vital Mind Reset, since it disburdens your system psychologically and physically. When you send your nervous system a signal of safety, you're able to make more empowered, true-to-you choices.

The next step is titration (baby steps) into teaching your system that the here and now is safe.

Only from your strong *No* can you bite into the juicy pear of your deepest *Yes*. As such, I'd like to offer a collection of self-containment hacks from which to select and practice, with diligent commitment, for *one week of your life*. These dedicated practices can lead to sustainable, self-sourced-safety.

Recapitulation

Featured in Taisha Abelar's book, *The Sorcerer's Crossing*, recapitulation is a shamanic practice intended to reclaim past energy.

The practice:

Make a list of your past sexual partners (you can also do this practice with any memories of any variety).

Sit and ground into the present by becoming aware of your feet on the floor, back, and seat.

Conjure up a memory of time spent with a past partner. With closed eyes, exhale and then turn your head to your right shoulder. Gaze across the scene as if you were witnessing it in real time, and then sweep your head to the left shoulder while inhaling your essence from the memory. Then, moving your head from your left shoulder to your right, exhale any energy that is not yours back into the scene.

Go back to the center, exhale again, and repeat several rounds until the memory fades. This is not a way to forget, but rather a means of collecting your *luminous cords* from the past to allow for memories to assemble without entanglements that drain your present-moment capacity to live and dream with intention.[6]

Replay your day before bed
Taking a minute to tidy up your memories can take a load off your psyche, so it doesn't have to process it all while you dream.

Lay down in bed, and before you drift off, let your mind think back on your day, in reverse chronological order. Start with your nighttime routine and finish with your first thoughts upon waking.

This kind of reflection will help you sort through and compartmentalize your experiences, and sometimes it will resolve feelings that you were too busy or overwhelmed to deal with in the moment, creating closure and thereby saving you from dreams filled with frustration.

Listen. Listen. Listen!
The immature masculine needs to fix, interrupt, and generally control the conversation. He's reactive, inattentive, and unobservant, and he's focused on what needs to change in order to feel okay.

Do *not* treat yourself this way!

Listen to yourself as if you're writing a dissertation on the story of your impulsive part, ashamed part, desperate part, resentful part, and scared part. Curiosity is the kingmaker in these lands, so when a protest arises within, don't talk yourself into safety and okayness, fake positivity, or distraction, or judge your inner critic with an even bigger critic.

Turn towards yourself and take thirty to ninety seconds to stop and actually listen to your internal voice the way you'd want to be listened to by your own loving, compassionate father or husband.

Create containers

Start practicing clear and intentional engagement.

When you are meeting with a friend, get clear on where, when, how long, and any financial desires (*Are we splitting the bill? Can I treat you tonight?*) that might take up emotional bandwidth to sort out in the moment.

Start by working with time, money, and general parameters that set you up for safety and comfort, verbalize that, and *stick to it*. Be the riverbanks to the water of your life.

Mature the Masculine Meditation

Five minutes is all you need to start this simple practice to help empty your mind and embrace silence.

Sit comfortably in a chair or on the floor, with your back straight, chin tucked, and spine long and straight, but not rigid. Relax your body, starting with the muscles of the face, neck, and shoulders, and then moving on to the rest of the body. Set your thoughts aside as you "set the intention to keep the mind clear."

Thoughts will come and go but keep your focus on allowing them to go without holding onto them or trying to remember them for later. This is about sitting with the thoughts and letting them pass through without gaining a foothold on your consciousness. Observe them without judgment, and softly allow your attention to rest in the spaces *between* those thoughts. You'll notice the brief time between one thought leaving and the next one entering is calm, peaceful, and quietly wide open, asking nothing, demanding nothing, just *there*.

It's okay if you can't spend much time in the space between your thoughts when you first try. With practice, that welcoming expanse will become an old friend, and you'll be able to spend more time there effortlessly. When you're done chilling in the twilight zone between thoughts, release your goal of clear mind, and allow your attention to return to your own energy. Become aware of how much calmer and more present you are once you've quieted the internal chatter and allowed yourself some time in the voids within your mind.[7]

Vampire breath

Bypassing spiritual pain with sunshine and rainbows isn't the path to alchemy. Amazingly, we have the capacity to ingest our so-called negative energies (from self or other) and transmute them to vital force. In this exercise, inspired by a book entitled *Vampire's Way to Psychic Self Defense*, we reclaim energy in its pure essence rather than labeling it as good or bad.

This exercise has 3 parts: Breath, Visualization, and Affirmation.

For the breathing part, find a comfortable position in a calm space and breathe tightly into the lower triangle of your abdomen. Think of it like a cauldron, and as you breathe in, instead of expanding the belly, you're contracting it along with your chest, creating a vacuum-like sensation in your core.

Now, imagine that all those big feelings you're having—the shame, disgust, anger, fear, rage—are a dark cloud of dust particles. Imagine that your breath is taking them all into that cauldron low in your belly. Then, hold that breath in, and think or say something self-assertive:

> *I call my power back.*
> *I am alive.*
> *I am impenetrable.*

Exhale and visualize that energy uncoiling from your lower belly, and as you allow it to rise up into your chest and heart, claim it as yours. Transmute that anger, fear, and rage into vital life force and use it to feed your soul. Call that energy back to yourself, knowing you have the capacity to hold aliveness in your system.[8]

Honor your boundaries
Boundaries aren't about pushing people away, demanding that they modify behavior, or making threats to get some distance; they're a way to honor yourself and others. Many times, we *think* we're speaking our boundaries, but instead we're actually letting our inner victims do the talking, often by over-explaining or diluting boundaries.

Here are a few simple, clear, non-confrontational phrases to use to express your *No*:

> *I'm not available for . . .*
> *This doesn't work for me.*
> *I'll consider it.*
> *You might be right.*

These are complete statements that will allow you to express a limit on what you're willing to engage in without falling into the jabbering validation explanation that makes saying "no" so awkward and uncomfortable. A healthy "no" shouldn't drive the right people away, either, and maintains regard, respect, and connection. Which leads me to something game-changing my erotic coach Whitney taught me:

The Appreciation Burrito

If the whole of something is mostly good, but there are aspects you don't want or can't accept, the appreciation burrito is a template for gentle constructive feedback. The layers of the burrito work like this:

Start with telling someone what you appreciate and what *is* working in a given situation, creating a safe space with you. Next comes the feedback, the problem, request, or trigger that made this little burrito necessary. Use "I statements" when possible, try to be clear and non-reactive, and avoid over-explaining. Finally, wrap this burrito up with even more delicious appreciation and gratitude. This way, your ask can be from the heart.

In the end, boundaries help you to be the keeper of your own heart and your own narrative and are a means of saying *Yes* to what becomes available through a *No*. If you've got you, and you know what you need and what works for you, then your choices are what keep you safe, and your embodied feelings will show you exactly what you need to know about your boundaries and your associated preferences.

Many of us are seeking a feeling of wholeness from a love that self-generates from deep within and is not contingent on the outside world. To get there, we must choose to reunite with our own bodies, feel all the feelings, and honor and release the stories that paper our prison walls. Because the truth is that we came here to experience it all, and you are ready when you are ready, and not a moment sooner. I suspect, however, that your moment may be now . . .

CHAPTER 8

Enter Through the Upset

Living Behind a Glass Wall

"Are you serious?!" I gasped that one fateful day my publicist called to tell me my first book had somehow made the *New York Times* bestseller list after a full mainstream media blacklisting. I remember it so vividly; I was on my cordless landline phone in my Manhattan office, and a surge of full-blown exhilaration came crashing over me. While this feeling invoked a sense of immediate excitement and energy, it lasted a mere thirty to sixty seconds before there was *nothing* left in its wake. True story: I felt nothing.

It was akin to a clitoral sneeze of an orgasm: a superficial sensation with no root system and no place to live inside my body. Why couldn't I celebrate this incredible accomplishment? I had built my whole life around full-on masculine achievement, reaching my so-called "goal" of climbing to the next rung of the ladder, and somehow there always seemed to be another rung that appeared just as I thought I was arriving at the top.

While this may seem like an extreme example, I'm sure you've felt the sense of inevitable, and yet surprising, emptiness that comes from masculine achievement and the product of your *doing-ness*. You get the grade, the promotion, the acceptance to the program, the book deal, the 10k (100k, million dollar) launch is yours, and . . . it just kind of feels about as thrilling as a new dress you wear out to dinner and then jam into your overstuffed closet, never to be sported again. Once you actually achieve the thing you've been tirelessly persevering over, it feels hollow. As a result, some of the most seemingly exalted moments in your life can feel utterly incomplete. I like to call this phenomenon "living behind a glass wall."

I remember distinctly, right around the time I started showcasing the work I do now, sitting down with a healer for a Body Talk session. In an effort to summarize my chief complaint, I said to her, "I have so many reasons to be happy; why does it feel like I'm living behind a glass wall?" It's like happiness is happening over there, and yet I'm still here, living in this narrow band of emotion. I might have been breaking glass ceilings, but the glass wall wasn't budging.

Know the feeling?

When's the last time you got what you really, really wanted, dear reader?

Did you relish and take in the exquisite feeling of havingness?

Or did you go right on keeping on, finding a new goal, or something else to worry about, complain about, or even someone to villainize mere moments later?

The plot twist, that we all know but easily forget, is that fulfillment doesn't come from having all the things, achieving all that's measurable, from everything working out, or even from manifesting what you *think* you most want. In my book, authenticity, and the permission to be alive, in our own skin, as we are, is what we're really after. And we can offer ourselves that permission, one pattern disruptor at a time.

The ultimate pattern disrupt is being with your sensations, turning toward your feelings, and creating space, even just a little, for them to be attended to with care. When you're in your masculine shell programs and defenses, you just don't do that. You avoid, fix, and suppress. But now, you will, by making a mantra out of this phrase: *enter through the upset.*

The No That You Already Know
Because Women Know Things

"What is something about your experience in your life that you know that you deeply wish you didn't know?" Adyashanti's words hung in the air of the vipassana room where the silence was so deep I could hear a pin drop. I allowed this question to drip deep into my psyche, where it would live forever as the single most incisive point of inquiry available to me and the women I serve. This inquiry illuminates the inner split, the part that knows and the part that does not want to know, and it's your job to introduce them to one another and divine a consensus between them. Answering this question will help you develop a deeper relationship to what you already know is a *No* for you, *and* you do not have to take action on it right away.

When I asked myself this question, I got to see how I continued to hold victim consciousness inside myself, and how I was indeed insisting that something in my reality "work" when it simply wasn't working, and *I knew it*. The answers that bubbled up for me took three years to manifest into reality, but the seeds of irreversible awareness were planted that day.

Patience with your own readiness and meeting yourself where you are is the feminine expression of trusting your process, knowing that there's divine timing and that you're not going to force yourself to be ready until you are. Indeed, readiness is the ephemeral moment when change feels more like *relief* than *terror*.

> **Go ahead . . . drop in, and ask it to yourself right now:**
> - *"What is something about your experience in your life that you know that you deeply wish you didn't know?"*
> - *Are you drinking too much coffee?*
> - *Is it time to have that conversation with your mother?*
> - *Are you stepping on the scale more often than feels good?*
> - *Is the whole work/mom balance thing just not work/mom balancing?*
> - *Are you simply not attracted to him anymore?*

You'll likely discover responses to this question *immediately* bubble up from within, the kinds of things that make you think, *Thank God I don't have to tell anybody about this!* It's like a secret confession between you and you. When you pose this question to yourself, in the privacy of your own mind, your inner defenders who are charged with explaining why you are persisting in a futile habit, pattern, or dynamic, get to rest for a moment so you can see more clearly where your energy is kinked up. Your answers might make you wince and cringe. It's important to remember that the wincing and cringing parts are there to protect you from the pain and shame of doing life wrong, and more precisely the rejection that might result. Beneath all these parts is a longing, unmet, awaiting your sacred gaze.

Enter Through the Upset

Rather than insist that something work when it simply doesn't, you can choose to feel what it's like to be forsaken, disappointed, frustrated, confused, hurt, and, in being with that inner experience, clarity will be delivered through self-devotion.

When you commit to entering through the upset, every so-called bad experience becomes an opportunity for alchemy. Whether someone cuts in front of you at the grocery store, iPhone rolls out a new track-and-trace feature, your daughter won't stop saying *Mama, mama, mama . . . look at this!*, and your husband watches TV on the couch while you tackle your resentment *and* all the essential household to-dos, or your boss's gaze lingers too long on your cleavage . . . whatever the hot spot is in your life: that's great! Lean into it with curiosity. I promise it's worth it. Your pain points are portals to inner alchemy. If you're only able to bypass or distract from your upset, if you constantly need to soothe and feel better, *you're not doing alchemy; you're doing allopathy.* Which means you're missing out on the richness of how you become the enchantress of your life. Instead, if you can stop everything for thirty seconds to three minutes when you first feel upset and *just* relate to your upset, you will radically shift your lifescape. Feel whatever's coming up, be with it, sit with it. Allow and approve of what's happening within your body. Become deeply interested and invested in yourself, openly and without judgment, story, or anything but simple attention offered to the sensation in your body.

This is a learned practice that begins with a fierce commitment to yourself and to the inherent meaning in your upset so that you can begin to create the conditions for your feelings to have a proper seat at your table (rather than banging down the door or cowering in the closet). This practice is storyless; it doesn't come with a litigation-level argument for why you should or shouldn't feel the way you do. It's simply a witnessing, and from that place you can choose how to interact with what is actually happening, without flying into the future or probing the past. Entering through the upset means you take every opportunity that upsets you to hone your skills as a deeply empowered woman. It means that whenever your specific victim story surfaces, you have a chance to expose, and ultimately evolve, these inner dynamics. And the beauty is that it doesn't take long.

Most of us do not experience the natural arc of emotional energy because, as children, we were told to calm down, stop crying, or gas-lit with "you're okay" when we clearly weren't. We grow up to imagine that if we start crying, we might never stop, because we never found out that tears begin, they peak, they resolve, and then they often turn into relief, laughter, or even pleasure. So, let's see where your arc takes you . . .

RECLAMATION REMEDY: ENTER THROUGH THE UPSET

Your #1 Practice
Feel The Feels

105

Some days just really grind your gears; your emotions are high, triggers are strong, and your reactions seem out of this world. Sometimes, all it takes is a breach in traffic etiquette, a perceived dis at work, or even just someone chewing a little too loudly, and you're off like a raging forest fire, ready to burn it all to the ground. Now, you can combust in this inferno of inflamed emotions. You can squash them down, stomp them out, or even intellectual-ize them so you can distance yourself through rigorous analysis . . .

Or (and this is the one I'm going to recommend) you can build a safe container for your feelings and allow yourself to *feel* them. That's right, actually *feel* those feels. And not because that's what a good woman does or because that's how to get them to go away. You choose to feel them simply because they are a part of *you*. **You are not your feelings; they are held by a part of you.** But your

---

feelings show you where there's room to acknowledge, listen, and witness.

Feel the Feels Success Tips
- Set a timer during this process, a type of self-husbanding that offers loving boundaries to your inner wild. Start with thirty to ninety seconds and work up to ten minutes.
- Do this in a comfortable space where you can feel safe to open up and be vulnerable. If you have to pull over in your car, take a private minute in the bathroom, or can actually take some time to lie down and focus on your body, remove yourself from the flow of life for the practice.

Now, conjure up the sensations and pay attention to where they show up. Enter into the sensation like a room, allow it to expand, even if it expands beyond the boundaries of your body. Breathe and *feel*.

Where do you feel it in your body?
Is it in your chest, like tight anxiety?
Can you feel it in your throat, like unspoken injustice?
Is it deep in your belly, where intuition resides?
Do you feel a weight on your shoulders?
Does it have a shape? A color? A taste?
What does it have to tell you?
Can you sit with it, and allow it to be, without running from it?
Can you let it get even bigger, beyond the bounds of your form?
Can you walk into the room of this feeling?

Become the masculine container that wholly loves and accepts everything you're feeling. As David Deida says, "Love your constricted throat," and stay open to what it tells you, instead of collapsing under the fear of how it can destroy you. The secret lies in surrender and true, loving acceptance. Open and allow. Open and allow.

Pendulating and Orienting into Your Feeling States
If it starts to feel a little too much, use Pendulation and Orienting to stay with what's arisen. These Somatic Experiencing practices, developed by Peter Levine and shared with me by my coach Whitney Lowery, are intended to resource your system enough so that you can face something uncomfortable without overwhelm and destabilization. As you Pendulate, your awareness encompasses more of the ecosystem of the body, and the charge may naturally lessen because you're no longer as desperate to get away from the sensation, push it away, or clench down around it to protect yourself.

Here's how to play with Pendulation and Orientation:

1. **Charge in the Chest, Stomach, or Throat:**
   Grab a pillow, a pet, or a soft object you can cuddle in your lap or hug tightly if needed. Take a moment to notice the sensation with just that small comfort item. Next, make the sound "voo" or any sound that feels soothing to you. Experiment. Some women prefer aaahs, uhhhs or ohms, and it might be helpful to play with different sounds to see what your body prefers right now.

   Then, sit in the stillness with natural, slow breaths, and notice if it's easier to be with your body and the sensations of the charge. Breathe and voo up to three times, as your attention swings back and forth between the charge and how it feels to voo.

2. **Charge in the Head, Neck, and Jaw:**
   Prop your elbows on something supportive and drop your face into your hands, allowing your neck to surrender its burden for a minute. Now, slowly open your mouth one to two inches and then close

107

it, gently and without tension. Notice what happens to the feeling as you let your powerhouse jaw muscles take a mindful break. Experiment with gently contorting your face, tensing (without biting down) and releasing the muscles to see if this makes it easier to focus on your face and neck.

3. **Charge in the Back, Arms, and Hands:**
As you take a deep breath into your belly, extend your arms fully, stretching your fingers out. Now, slowly, so slowly, curl those fingers in, one by one, until you've formed two tight fists. Feel the sensations from your fingertips, through your arms, to your face. Once fully clenched, slowly open them, relax, and allow your arms to hang limp. Notice how the charge responds to tensing and relaxing your hands and arms.

4. **Charge in the Legs, Feet, Buttocks, Hips, and Pelvis:**
As you take a deep breath, lift one foot off the ground about three inches. Pause to notice the sensations of this position, and how these new sensations might be mixing with the charge; feel the leg-lift and the charge simultaneously. On an exhale, let the foot drop. Notice the difference between your legs. For symmetry, stand up, then sit back down. Has the charge dispersed some so that it's not so condensed in one place?

5. **Full Body Charge that Feels Numbing or Too Big:**
For this practice, gently press a pillow to your belly or lap, and sense your body's response. Is it comforting to feel the contact of the pillow? If not, put the pillow away. With your shoes off, place your feet flat on the ground and wiggle your toes to wake up sensation. Slowly and gently, let your eyes focus on something in your environment that is pleasant

and calming to look at, and observe any relief or pleasure in your body. Allow your attention to swing back and forth between the charge and the comfort you feel by looking at something beautiful. Is this making it easier to stay with sensation and feel the feels?

Sometimes, when digging into these big feels, you can activate your system's fight response. That's okay, and this is a great time to work on upping your own resilience and capacity to deal with those emotions by processing them in smaller doses. Here are a couple ways you can cater to your fight response without going out and joining a Fight Club:

- "Combining a voo with a growl." Voo deeply from your belly, then let your face become a snarl as you softly let that voo become a growl, stretching your jaw and activating your brows. You can even get on your hands and knees, really feeling the sensations and vibrations of the voo and the facial muscles' expression of rage, fight, anger, and predatory power.
- Get on all fours and play with being a wild, ferocious beast self. A lioness, a she-wolf, a great bear— embody the animal, slowly scratching, growling, articulating every movement as your spine snakes, your hips circle, and your teeth bare. The magic is in the embodiment and the slow expression of your actions, so your attention is on the feelings, not the story behind the feelings. You're thinking about the fierceness of the animal, capable of fighting and defending, as you rock back and forth, feeling the weight on your wrists and hands, in your knees and feet.
- If you can express anger without adding to the story that created the emotion, you can clear that feeling by giving action to the urges. We're talented at talking about why we feel something, but what about

109

communicating what you're feeling non-verbally? Punch a pillow, kick the air, rail at the sky! But do it at 50 percent intensity so that you can feel the subtler sensations of whatever you're doing. For example, when you punch, feel it from your fingers to your face to your feet. More intensity may seem more cathartic, but don't mistake exhaustion for release.

- Bite it out! The jaw is a powerhouse of stored tension, and sometimes the best way to release it is to lean in. You can get a strong piece of leather, a particularly sturdy pillow, even some super tough jerky, and work those jaw muscles by clenching them about 10 percent more at a time, taking care of your teeth, and experimenting with adding more tension and then relaxing the tension. Notice how the sensations in your jaw change as you consciously clench and release.

- If the punching and kicking feels good, try slowing it down. Like you're fighting in a giant jar of honey, slow down your movements and fully express each gesture. As you curl your fist, extend your arm, and push, punch, or kick something away from you, slow it down and notice the muscles and physical sensations of the action. To explore further, focus on softening everything after the gesture. How do the feelings change as you unclench your jaw, soften your belly, and drop your shoulders? Does your breath impact these sensations?

- As anger often masks feelings of powerlessness, it's important to let yourself explore what lives behind and beneath the feelings of rage. Try to get soft, drop down, and let those feelings come in like "I lost" or "I wasn't strong," or "I need help" and let yourself settle into this tender, vulnerable place. Notice if you're tensing against that tenderness to protect yourself. Soften your eyes, jaw, and shoulders, un-brace your belly and breathe, and when you feel more physically relaxed, revisit the place with the most sensation.

- Vocalize the unspoken. We bite our tongues for the comfort of others. This is when you take a minute to express yourself, raw and unfiltered. Say a thing, then notice where you feel it in your body. Say another thing and allow yourself to be with the embodied experience. Spit venom, then feel. Speak hatred or rage, then *feel*. Let it all out, in a landslide of unfiltered verbal vitriol. Slow it down and let yourself be with your body as you take time to give voice to those thoughts and feelings knowing they are just a narrative held by a part.[1]

Short on time? Check out the . . .
Down & Dirty Feel the Feels Practice:
This practice doesn't have to take you completely out of your day; in fact, it's designed to be integrated into your life!

Any time you get a little hint of upset, you can literally stop what you're doing, go to the bathroom or to your car, set a thirty-second timer, and just see:

Where do I feel this?

Rather than sitting and thoroughly exploring the entirety of sensation, this practice is meant to allow you to honor whatever the feelings want to say. By expanding the permission field, allowing and accepting the feelings, you'll finally alchemize what those feelings are attached to.

So, feel the feels, thank them for their messages, and then let them pass through without causing an internal natural disaster along the way.

Through self-relating and self-intimacy, you turn toward the discomfort within and say: *I'm here, I'm interested, and I fundamentally welcome whatever is into the space, without judging.* An important nuance is to remember the intention to *be with what is* rather than offering support, positive affirmations, or reassurance to the part that is feeling the tough feelings. This also happens to be a Victimless Mothering tip when it comes to relating to your children. Get curious and listen rather than convincing, coercing, or "educating."

I remember looking out over my backyard a year or so ago and taking in the beauty of the filtered light, the banyans, my chickens, and the sound of water trickling. The air was the perfect temperature, and my afternoon was mine to play with. I became aware of a deep ache of loneliness. Almost immediately, an inner voice piped up that said, *no need to feel lonely! You have your friends over often, you're seeing your girls tonight, and don't forget your kitties!* This voice, of course, comes from a well-meaning "protector" charged with keeping difficult feelings like loneliness under wraps. Thank you, protector! But to allow the lonely feeling to simply be, grow, expand, and belong requires that a mature adult witness hold that space. That's exactly what your intention can offer.

Your Weapon as a Woman (And What Happens When You Wield it)

In the realm of man-woman relating, you will encounter your victim story when you're attempting to source love and connection from an impossible place, insisting that what's in front of you *must, can, and should* be different than it is. In these moments, it's easy to get swept up in old imprints and wage an inner war on an outer battlefield because you can't clearly see, let alone accept, what's in front of you. When our old (or even lineage-level ancient) wounds get reactivated, the last thing most of us want to do is reveal our feminine heart in vulnerability. The truth (and irony) is that when you feel rejected, betrayed, or afraid, you're often craving connection, but are likely to create the very circumstances for the familiar disconnection of your childhood.

In the personalized menu of fight, flight, freeze, and fawn stress physiology, a woman's fight response to unsafety is her capacity to shame men. Leveraging the essential value of his status and reputation, she unsheathes her sword and spares no dimension of his self-concept. In fact, a woman's socially decimating capacity to shame is the counterpart to a man's capacity to literally kill. When we have the impulse to frame a perceived source of injury as bad and wrong, we may tap into this age-old arsenal and mount a case for why *we* are right and how irreparably damaged *he* is. We'll recruit half a dozen girlfriends as well-led jurors and the prosecution begins. Reputation destruction is a high art in some circles of hens.

I like to think that my soul consented to and architected my cardinal wounds, and I now have the power of choice in assigning them meaning. Every time your wounds get activated, you're presented with a fork in the road: to either enter through the upset so you can be with the felt experience, connect to your vulnerability, and attend to yourself in order to make wise choices, or engage your familiar patterns and even litigate around your upset from the lens of superiority. I now *know* when I am choosing the well-trodden path and when I'm ready to take those ninety seconds so that I can step onto the road less traveled.

Over my years as a professional provocateur, I've had *several* experiences of being rejected from communities for my beliefs and behaviors. I've been rejected for my health beliefs, scientific stance, and I've even been uninvited from a wedding because of my perspective on plandemic mandates. I *know* what it is to be rejected for my mind, and these days I actually find it entertaining. However, since I have decided to express what feels good in my body, highlight what brings me joy, and de-secret aspects of my sexuality to the world, I have encountered *massive* amounts of shame that says, *stop! You're doing it*—being a woman—*wrong!* One such instance arose when I was removed from a membership that espouses Christian values—at the specific behest of several members—for my public demonstrations of so-called "immodesty," "promiscuity," and "profanity." While I do not identify with any denominational religion, I absolutely support and live by the ethos of many of the values central to this online community.

When I received the email about my removal, I felt a slight eleva-tion of my heart rate, a wave of heat going up my neck, and the urgent impulse to pen a response. I felt it my duty to show them how wrong they were about me and about their decision, and then, for good measure, about their perspectives on immodesty, promiscuity, and profanity. Instead of attending to myself, I wrote and sent a playful but pedantic and pretty damn condescending email. I am frequently applauded for *slaying* the email with rhetorical eloquence, precision, and surgical-level shaming capacity, but in this instance, the woman who called me to the carpet was my erotic coach, Whitney Lowery.

In her classical fierce compassionate energy, Whitney reminded me that there were *so* many ways I was enacting and embodying that which I was judging, and that I seemed to be in my shadow habit of trying to educate someone out of their ignorance. She reminded me that if someone doesn't ask to be educated, they probably don't want to be.

Celebratory sidenote: In the old days of my incarnation, I would not have had any awareness that I was jumping into my pattern of immediately responding and trying to get them to *see* (nor would I have sent the follow up apology email that I dispatched after I came to). Now my somatic sequence is familiar. I feel a clenching in my chest, I feel heat waves move under my arms and up my neck, and these sensations are attended by the impulse to defend and protect myself. In this particular scenario, I had perceived a small *No* and a whisper that said, *there's another way,* and I had a sneaking suspicion I really could be doing better by now, and yet, I still hit *send*. And by so doing, I abandoned the part of me who was *asking* me for my own attention. That shame-triggered somatic sequence in my chest and throat was the gatekeeper, redirecting me to action so that I could preserve social status and a sense of righteousness. Had I chosen to pause and allow the shame to wash over me and my body to take its curled shape, it's possible that I might have felt a flash of anger, a clench of shame, a flare of fear, and then likely tears of sadness. The alchemical arc of the feelings would have been engaged, and I would

114

have ridden it to clarity and creativity, while reuniting my consciousness and my heart.

By leaning into my "I'll get them to see" stance, I was abandoning the part of myself that was holding the *feelings* about the rejection so that I could focus on "fixing" what was outside of me. So, as often happens when our core wounds get activated, I was trying to source from an impossible place, seeking to create connection and safety while resolving an inner conflict, when none of these things were ever on offer from this place. And when we are honest with ourselves, we know from the start whether something is a fit for our needs. We know because we are women and we sense these things in our bones, in our hearts, in our pussies. We feel a little *yes* or a little *no,* and this sensed navigational cue tells us whether something is for us. The moment I received that email, I saw who and what I was dealing with and the fundamental incompatibility at play. It was a little, *nope, this isn't for you, Kelly.* And to have honored and aligned with that would have given me the opportunity to also align with my tender parts. Luckily, there will always be another opportunity to master self-allegiance . . .

As a reminder, connection with yourself (and others) is not available from a place of superiority, which often looks like a litigation-level diatribe that demonstrates *all* the reasons you think you're completely right about how your husband, boss, or intended email recipient is dead wrong. Your attempt to secure just a little sense of okayness in a sea of felt wrongness will never change anyone, and it will only further fracture your inner mosaic. It never feels good because what we *really* want is connection, and the little voice inside is usually saying something like, *I'm afraid you don't love me, and I'll never be lovable.*

The remarkable thing is that you can never go wrong by revealing your feelings from a place of vulnerability. In contrast to feminine directives, the truth is that few things are more beautiful than a woman embodying vulnerability. By expressing how you actually felt about something (*I felt ashamed*), or even sharing the raw emotion with a gasp or an ouch, and then taking *responsibility* for your lived and felt experience, you can discover the sense of *rightness* that you've been seeking through your habitual victim-triangle style of behavior.

When you align with felt experiences, you see what is truly wanted, and you can ask, or you can offer. Most of the time, we will offer/ask in a mushy mixed bag that makes no one feel good. When you're *offering* education, insights, or time ("If you'd like to speak about this, I'm available,") when it's something you actually *want*, you are self-betraying. If asking for what you want would sound more like, "I want you to make me feel better, include me, like me," then odds are, you'd recognize that all of that is your responsibility, and then there's no email, text, or message to send at all. Just an opportunity for you to be with you.

When you come into alignment with your feelings and practice deep self-allegiance, you'll be able to hold your power of choice close to your heart, and you will no longer need to make anyone bad and wrong to orient towards what you really want.

You want to leave your relationship? You want to quit your job? Move your body from one side of the room to the other? You simply do it; it's your *choice*. You don't have to make a big campaign about why that thing sucks, or how it harmed you, or parade around phrases like, "He was such a narcissist" in order to be legitimized in what it is that you want and boldly align with what is right for you.

CHAPTER 9

Villain Crown: Own Your Badness

Meet your Medusa

I don't know about you, but I've always suspected that there was a part of me that was completely unlovable, right to the core. And then I met her.

One fall afternoon during a *powerful* self-led ceremony, I felt like I was seated around a campfire listening to a mythical tale. I was introduced to a Medusa character, and it was revealed that she was the antagonist in the story of my life. The twist at the end of the tale, however, was that this villainous Medusa, this despicable and "evil" enemy, actually lived *inside* of me, and, inexplicably, *was* me. The medicine journey revealed that I have incarnated to hold, *very specifically*, the Medusa archetype. Now let's get this straight: this wasn't the pseudo-sexy, wild-woman Medusa with perfect perky green breasts and sensually writhing snake hair you might have seen in a music video. No, this Medusa was an ugly witch of a she-beast, striking terror into everyone who crosses her path. She is *thoroughly* un-huggable, not cute, and isolated beyond all measure.

It became starkly clear to me that any desirable superficial trappings that I might possess were merely on loan to me as a part of my incarnation's soul mission: *to reclaim the dark power of women for women and men alike*. In order to fulfill this mission, I was given the Trojan Horse of an outwardly attractive appearance so that I could move beyond the margins of society and "into the walls of the palace," so to speak.

This reveal of my core inner dark Self seemed to resolve decades of dissonance and explain why I have often felt terrified that I would be exposed as crazy, ugly, or otherwise too horrible to love. I've (half) joked that I hustled to earn my place on the *right* side of the psychiatrist's desk so no one would know that *I'm* the crazy one. Meeting my Medusa demystified why I've believed, to my core, that when I am fully expressed I had better be prepared to be alone forever, because *nobody* wants that. *No one* can handle that. No *man* can handle me. Thus, I will be left alone, bereft and forsaken by all but my cats and chickens.

The ensuing opportunity became learning how to see, understand, and love my inner Medusa, to perhaps even find others who specifically love me not in spite of but *because* of this core essence (just like the king in "The Handless Maiden" who loves the forested woman in all her wild pear juice-covered glory). Because, like Russian dolls, inside of this inner dark witch dimension of me lives a tender, sweet child that she cares for and loves.

As with all reclamation journeys, to love your most unlovable parts starts with you, and it doesn't start with love, per se: it starts with intention and attention.

This chapter is designed to empower you to meet the monsters in your mirror. This is where, in the feel it, face it, free it order of operations, we practice *facing* our inner monstress. And instead of looking away as fast as you can, your invitation is to fully take in your monstrosity for all her majesty. This step is the truce; it's the end of the war and the beginning of the symphony that can only be conducted when enough bass is invited into the room.

We'll start by introducing you to your "villain crown," probing the ways you've learned that it's safer to project your shadows onto others, so that you can fully handle and play into the holofractal nature of Self, feeling into and befriending all the pieces of you you've pushed away behind that old shamewall.

It's time to coronate yourself, woman!

Villain Crown

Villainy is out these days. As virtue signaling has made its way into "public health," sex and race relations, and college campus microaggression management, we are a sea of entitled victims, finger pointing the bad guy, hoping Mommy Medicine and Daddy Government lend their approval. What happened to the wicked witch and evil queen? The ruthless tyrant? It's time to reclaim that archetype because we're already playing in it. Remember that the victim triangle roles are fluid, and she who seems the villain may actually be the savior of your soul, inducing the growth and reclamation that would never otherwise be available, and he who plays the victim or savior is often a villain to someone else. Beauty is in the eye of the beholder, after all.

Steeped in New Age pacifist programming, it took a lot for me to even perceive the part of me that is the punisher. The part of me that can only be described as a vicious bitch. I'm talking about a cutting, slaying, *I will fuck you up* part of me. She's well-cloaked and stands right behind the more palatable savior here to right the wrongs of society and vanquish the enemies of freedom and truth. And because my girlfriends and I practice taking personal responsibility, plumbing the depths of our struggles for meaning, and minimizing the open mic time our victim parts are allowed, the punisher isn't really invited to our gatherings.

She's in there. I believe she's in each of us. That destroyer, that slayer, that wild, raw, awe-inspiring Cruella. But we pretend she's not, and so all she gets is a few sideways moments of whiny complaint or a frustrated harumph when we are triggered. She is well-corralled by shame because she's not allowed to exist, according to the societal rules we've consented to.

But what if she holds the keys to a deep dimension of feminine eros? The power of this shame alchemy lies in the fact that most of us are terrified of soulful, dark feminine sexuality. Men are terrified to fall under the spell of the seductress, and women are terrified that they'll be burned at the stake if they're branded one. So, we hide our darkness, our sexuality, our badness, and we live half-alive.

Amazingly, your imagination, your creative energy, your aliveness *is* your sexual energy. So is your wild energy, your angry energy, your destructive energy, your "enough is enough" energy. We fail to recruit our native power in service of the creation of our life, *because* we are not well-apprenticed in how to work with it. If you are afraid of the orgasm that will dissolve you into the state of annihilation, if you're afraid of your scream, of your ugly cry, of the energy of your unfettered *fuck No*, you are only accessing a sliver of your audacious energy.

Heart-connected dark feminine erotic power has the capacity to destroy what needs to go. This is the primordial *No* that reduces all the trash to compost and transforms it into fertility. In this creative space, new life springs forth just over the threshold of death and loss. The dark feminine sees and knows the unsavory truth of what's in front of her.

The Reclamation of your inner darkness is a big one. In some ways, it's *the* big one. It's the practice of alchemizing the single greatest drain on your energy (shame) into the birthright of your existence as a human (creativity) that will bring you home to your feminine power.

There are three ways to practice wearing the villain crown:

1. When others judge you
2. When you judge others
3. When you worry that sex is taking up too much or too little of your lifescape

Putting on your villain crown is all about getting comfortable with being the bad girl, the antagonist, the dark witch, the unwanted, the soiled, the reckless, the tainted in someone else's eyes. It's about allowing other people to have their perspectives and opinions, thus resolving endless efforts toward reputation management and trying to share a reality with every person you meet.

When you get to the place where you can simply *be* the bad character in the film of your life or in someone else's script, you free up a treasure trove of beautiful bandwidth to focus on what you want to create. You get to focus on life's more expansive questions like: *What do I want to give my energy to? What really lights me up? What do I actually want???* Which is so much more pleasurable than micromanaging things you can't control—i.e., other people's opinions of you!

VILLAIN CROWN INVENTORY: WHERE IS YOUR GOOD GIRL STORY OWNING YOU?

There's a saying that when two people meet, there are actually six people involved.

For each person, there are three facets of themselves: there's how they see themselves, there's how they're seen by the other person, and there's who they truly are.

Take a moment to think about what that means for any given relationship.

For every aspect of yourself that you wish you could change, or know that others might reject if they knew, there's often a pattern of behavior you adopt to help offset some of those shadows. To put it a little more bluntly: sometimes you act like a fake AF good girl so other people will like you more. This appeasement strategy has a very good track record and does work . . . until our inner parts start to rattle the gilded cage.

By spending so much effort managing others' opinions of you, you self-abandon and can even create a fracture where you believe the lie, only to be hair-triggered when the reality of your shadow side gets called out. A harmonious life comes when you can reconcile the cognitive dissonance of all three facets of your being into one honest, cohesive whole. That way, when you meet other people, it's authentically as yourself, not some clumsily curated projection of who you think will secure connection, approval, and "good and right girl" status.

Take a minute to really consider your good girl story:

What is the one criticism that would absolutely decimate you?
What is a nice or kind thing you do or have done, and how would it feel if you were criticized or judged for your intentions?
Do you ever give time, attention, energy, or gifts and feel unappreciated?
What kind of woman do you feel represents the biggest problem in society right now?

Take a moment to really *be* with your answers. What do you notice in your body?

If you choose to follow your curiosity, you might realize there's a mirror here, waiting to show you the tiny little mirror inside all of us, because the things you judge most in others are often the things you try the hardest to hide about yourself—even from yourself!

Does that sting a little? It's nothing compared to the wallop you'll feel if your secrets are exposed without taking a moment to see and own the villain traits within.

What I've noticed is the universe prefers harmony, and until you do this shadow work, you'll attract those you most judge into your life as mirrors reflecting your unseen dimensions. Failure to own your villain will only leave you in a world of judgment, where you can only be "good" if others hold your bad.

RECLAMATION REMEDY: THE UNSPOKEN SCRIPT

We all have an unspoken script.

Like a caption banner that runs beneath every interaction and situation, a part of us is nobly tasked with narrating an inner experience that is often at odds with what we express on the outside. The thing is, this part wants the mic too, and it is sick of the appeaser always hogging the stage.

When you're exhausted from showing up to play nice, keep things moving, or otherwise feeling the heaviness of what is unexpressed, try this:

Set a timer for five minutes and write down every unspeakable, whiny, bitchy, complainy, unspiritual, shitty thing you have to say about a person or situation. If there were no consequences, and the world depended on this part's brutal self-expression, whatdya got? Let it rip and then burn it, flush it, or complete the catharsis by tearing it into a billion bits.

Know that you've honored something that is inside you, whether you like it or not.

Wear Your Crown Loud and Proud

"You are a deeply injured soul, incapable of love."

Those words hit me like a freight train. My stomach did approximately a hundred somersaults when I read the pixelated words on my screen, hovering at the top of a treacherous email from somebody that I cared very, very deeply about, and it was, of course, in a context of greater contention. Thankfully, once the initial shock subsided, and because I was practiced at entering through the upset and wearing my villain crown, I was able to fully explore that less than warm and fuzzy missive. I thought to myself: What if I didn't defend myself?

Not fully retired, my inner litigator wanted to come online and venomously respond as to why I'm so right, and the writer so wrong, using factual, throat-cutting defenses and evidence to underpin my case. But if there's anything I've learned through this work, it's that this comment was triggering and painful *because* a part of me agreed with this sentiment. So, I went in to meet that part. In the privacy of my home, I took her villain crown of badness and unlovability and rested it atop my curly brown locks. I looked in the mirror, I stood a bit straighter, and I tried on the accusations.

I am a deeply injured soul. I am incapable of love.

For those precious moments of seeming role play, I could get into character enough to own the truth in those statements. Deeply injured? Sure. Incapable of love? Well, I'm learning every day what love and secure attachment actually looks like. I had only started to learn how to love by collecting all the parts of myself that I hated, the parts that I would project outside of myself and fight with "out there." In fact, this whole book is about that very topic, so there must have been some work to do in that arena. So, sure, that too.

So, was this person in their right to cast these slanderous remarks? Sure. And it was this anticlimactic acknowledgement of these grains of truth held by parts of me I would rather have ignored that gave way for me to declare: "Okay, cool . . . moving on now." Sometimes you can really quite literally take the piss out of even the most intense criticism or soul-crushing comment by just trying it on and whispering to yourself, *maybe it's true . . .*

RECLAMATION REMEDY: PUT ON YOUR VILLAIN CROWN

Reminder: When someone, especially someone you care about, criticizes you, it only hurts because you recognize and identify with some part of their criticism, and deep down, you fundamentally agree with them. The next time someone throws shade and your nervous system overloads with shame and indignation, take a beat and wonder: *What's in this for me?*

When someone points the finger of judgment at you and labels you as "bad," try it on for size. I'm not saying make it your favorite outfit, but just see how it feels.

If someone calls you selfish, could you own that? The truth is: we all are. We are wired to meet our needs, directly or through seeming altruism. Ironically, when someone accuses you of selfishness, they are often saying "pay more attention to me" in classical "selfish" fashion.

If someone says you're being a superior bitch, take a minute to explore how you might, in fact, be a superior bitch. Or self-righteous jerk. Or narcissistic meanie.

124

What if they say you're being inappropriate? Reckless? Rude? Tone-deaf?

Can you let them have their own villain moment? Let them do their thing, finger point and judge, and see what self-discovery they've unwittingly gifted you. The truth is, they're probably embodying exactly what they say you're doing, so the mirror strikes again.

Play with saying accepting phrases out loud or privately in your head, like *"Maybe you're right,"* or *"Thanks for your opinion, I'll consider it."*

If you take the time to think about it, you might come to realize they're right, even if it's just a little bit. Even 5 percent right deserves some extra thought and integration.

Ask that protector part of you in open, curious inquiry: *What am I making it mean for that to be true?*

What am I making it mean to be dressed provocatively? What is a whore anyways, and what does their dress code have to do with how others see you?

What am I making it mean to be seen as needy and attention seeking? Why do I see needy as a bad thing, and when did this relationship with need start? How did I start believing I couldn't have needs and still be a "good girl"?

Make as few assumptions as possible and truly explore while allowing the feeling state to simply exist in your body.

Can you be with that part and develop curious intimacy? How can you listen to what that part has to say and not try to correct it, convert it, or spiritually bypass it into some sort of self-confident, self-validated space?

Simply give this part a seat at your table.

The Woman That You Judge: Hint, It's You!

When you really look deep into your dark feminine shadows and probe why you feel like you have to be the good girl, you'll likely discover that you don't want to acknowledge that you in fact feel superior to others, especially other women (and your exes).

Resolving superiority means putting to bed the tendency to put somebody down in order to feel okay about yourself, *especially* if that person is acting in ways you've decided that you don't. You might find that you need someone to be less haughty, less loud, less incompetent, less flakey, less flirty, less rude, less asleep, just *less* in order to feel right in yourself. This is a very unstable identity construct that is inevitably going to be challenged because your dark bits are living in those other women. This illusion of spiritual hierarchy runs rampant in the New Age, and even in the activist community, where we imagine that we are so much better than the so-called "sheep" out there who are completely asleep and painfully unaware of their patterns and programs. It fuels the enormous eye-roll where we delight in the judgment of the ones who aren't doing the "work," the plant medicine, who aren't cleaning up their motherline, who are (GASP!) eating gluten and using fluoridated toothpaste! Let alone the woman on her couch eating Cheetos, giving zero fucks about bettering herself or saving the world.

The problem is that this form of spiritual high-brow superiority means you can't authentically connect to others, and you are, naturally, projecting heaps of judgment onto an aspect of yourself while you do it. For me, this shows up as judging "lazy" or "incompetent" women. I am, in fact, pushing away a part of myself who wants to soften into her feminine and not be in full-on hyperdrive all the time, the part that wants help and support, and the part that wants to still be loved even if she's not useful.

Just as I've experienced judgment for my publicly disclosed pole dance journey, I too have judged women whom I imagined to be "hypersexual" (hyper relative to what?!), unprofessional, attention-seeking, and needy. I used to feel deeply envious of women who were speaking out publicly about the reclamation of eros (women whom I later showcased on my own platform, of course). Why does Mama Gena get to teach in a negligee? Why does Kim Anami get to say the words "fuck" and "cock"? And why does Sheila Kelley get to use pole dancing as a form of therapy while I "have to" be locked into this too-confining box of erudite scientist clinician? This protest lived underneath a subtle but real sense of being more legitimate and important than women who were showcasing sexual energy online. In fact, these women I judged and compared myself to were torch-bearers for me, revealing where I wanted to stretch and extend my own expression. Because underneath your judgment of other women, and your sense of superiority, lies a permission field to expand into womaning in a far more pleasurable, dimensional, and liberated way.

RECLAMATION REMEDY:
RESOLVE SUPERIORITY OVER YOUR MOTHER

Do you feel superior to your mother? Be honest. Emotionally, intellectually, physically, spiritually? I mean, you've done all this work, put in all this effort to heal, and now you "get it" so much more. That has to count for something. So maybe you do feel just a touch (or maybe a whole lot) of superiority.

But are you really, though?

How can you access the ways in which your mother needed to be exactly who she was (and is) in order for you to prioritize what matters so much to you today?

Ask yourself this: *How did your mother show you what you actually want for yourself in this lifetime?*
Did she model the type of woman you strive to be? Or did her behavior serve as a cautionary tale on how you *never* want to be? How did she play a role in creating the conditions for you to be clear about what works for you, what feels good, what you like and don't like?

And if you want to get metaphysical, is it possible that she signed up to be the unenlightened one so that you could feel what reclamation is actually like? I mean, would you even be reading this book if it wasn't for her? What if you're just two flavors of woman connected forever in the web of divinity?

Relatedly, how has your mother groomed you to access more and deeper shades of femininity?

When I look at my own motherline, I can clearly see the many archetypes the women who came before me have embodied. They were traditional women who upheld their place in the home, they worked hard, raised children. One took her own life, and another remained celibate for forty-plus years, but one thing I believe they all had in common is that they never danced. It's easy for me to feel superior for exploring this glorious facet of myself instead of hiding it away. Clearly, I'm more woman, more feminine, more aligned, right? But how did my mother and my mother's mother and my mother's mother's mother work to create the space, resources, and contrast I needed to explore this aspect of my own womanhood?

Coming from an Italian background, the women in my life were never stingy with their own judgments. Your hair is too dry, your lipstick is too loud, are you sure that shirt is enough shirt to go out in?

Big surprise that my own reclamation journey has staked bold claims on beauty, sensuality, and self-expression, when I experienced cautionary energy around being "too much." Most mothers want you to be authentically *who you are,* but they source safety by molding you in their own image. This is what psychology calls the narcissistic extension, where a parent can live their unlived lives through their children. I like to think that I live through my mother's unlived dreams of beautiful, sensual expression every time I dance, and that doesn't make me better than her. It just means she raised me to be *me,* and to reach for My Self with the core of my very being.

Think a minute on what resources and capacity your own mother had.

How much freedom did she have in her life to live her truth? How much opportunity was she given to reflect on her roles as a woman and to embody her own beliefs? And then look at what you have, and what opportunities you were given that she never was.

Feel your way into appreciation for the possibility that your mother was exactly who she was so that you can be exactly who you are.

True reclamation leaves these feelings of superiority behind, because no one individual knows how to woman better than any other, and you are only the expert on you.

THE WOMAN IN THE ROOM YOU JUDGE: SMOKE OUT THE SISTER WOUND SHADOW

Related to the mother wound is the perilous realm of woman-on-woman hate. We've all heard of the sisterhood of women, but I don't think a single one of us has escaped an all-girl event without a hint of side-eye, a whiff of judgment, or even a scathing encounter.

When comparison is a safety strategy, imagined superiority and inferiority relative to other women becomes a means of orienting. But those in glass houses shouldn't throw stones, right? In order to liberate yourself from the funhouse mirrors that distort your own fears back to you, you first need to recognize when you are in judgment of your sisters.

It's time to follow your humble curiosity and pay attention when you find yourself judging another woman in public. In fact, actively seek out the woman who rubs you the wrong way, for whatever reason. Maybe she's too brash, too flirty, too big with her movements and loud with her laughs. Or maybe she's too meek, too nice, too accommodating and ingratiating. Whatever it is, look around and check in to see if there's a reaction that feels viscerally ick in your body.

With an open mind, ask yourself:

What would you say to her if there were no social consequences?
What do you imagine would happen if you were more like her?
What would be the upside of being more like her?
What is the downside of being like yourself?
Is it possible there's a similar part inside yourself?
A way that you're just like her?

Explore the mirror she brazenly holds up for you. Is there any part of the current behavior you're exhibiting that is reminiscent of exactly what you're hating on? Like are you judging a sister for being aloof and cold while you ice-grill her from across the room?

Each of these rejected aspects of yourself and others are just waiting to give you the gift of self-insight and permission. May every woman that you judge help you meet a part of yourself that wants permission to be just like her.

When you see others as bad, why not lean into being the villain?
Think about what or who you hate, and why. Hate is a strong word, but it evokes victim stories, so let's play with it.

Write a scathing hate mail to the object of your derision:

- How do you want them to be punished? Get detailed.
- Get granular about why they are wrong and why you're judging them.
- Demand they admit that you are, in fact, right, and they should be sorry for ever being wrong.

We aren't sending this letter. This letter never needs to see the light of day. All it needs to see is a fireproof container and a match, because you're going to light this piece of hate literature on fire.

As you watch it burn, consider if there is any aspect of their loathsome behavior that you're currently embodying yourself? In other words, are you *irrationally expecting an irrational person to behave rationally, and then judging them for not being rational?*

Now let's integrate this exercise.
Take it back from the external lens and focus inside. Remember that the people you judge, criticize, and even downright *hate* are giving you a divine opportunity to sort through the attic of your own shit and discover the parts of yourself that are terrified of being guilty of what you actively condemn. Revel in the small hypocrisy and let it set you free.

One of the more delicious lessons I've learned through the act of wearing my villain crown is this: If women can commit to this one thing, *just this one thing*, the safety we long for may become available. I'm talking about this one thing: Stop imagining that you know how another woman should be womaning. You do not know better how another woman should be living her life, loving, dressing, and speaking. You're not the expert or authority; you only know about you. And if you think you know about her, odds are you don't even know about you.

So, stay in your lane. I'll stay in mine. And if we poke each other where it hurts, we'll enter through the upset, wear the villain crown, see if we're trying to buy eggs from the hardware store, and reclaim our power of choice.

You have choice, so you don't need to hate.
You have choice, so you don't need to condemn.
You have choice, so you don't need to be around anything that
*   doesn't work for you.*

And more importantly, you don't need this entity, this being, this situation to be *bad* and *wrong* in order to make a sovereign choice.

Victimless (And Villain-Free) Mothering: Breaking the Generational Cycle

Thus far, the down and dirtiest Villain Crown work I've done has been wearing the Villain Crown as a mother (that's when the tables really turn!). Because yes, we think we are superior to our mothers until we become mothers ourselves, and we confront that notorious fork in the road: defend your narrative or validate your child's lived experience. Perhaps because motherhood is the actualization of the woman in her life-giving power, to bear the weight of condemnation and failure cuts a layer too deep for most.

Through much of the re-parenting I have done of my own child self, I have learned to emotionally self-regulate, take personal responsibility, and empathically and non-defensively visit with my children's life experiences. Invested in my own narrative that I have ended many lineage-level cycles of abuse, disembodied self-betrayal, and addiction in my family line, I felt pretty confident that I was the adult child, and not the emotionally immature parent, when I opened Gibson's book *Adult Children of Emotionally Immature Parents*. So, one day, I felt inspired to ask my daughters two questions to support our deepening intimacy:

1. *What is something that I did that hurt you that, when you think about it now, still hurts you?*
2. *What do you need from me, these days, that I'm not giving you?*

Through this simple exercise, I was able to see how I too was at risk for experiencing my children as narcissistic extensions, meaning that my self-worth was contingent upon my agreement with their responses and their affirmation of my experience. What if they reflected something other than "Mama, you've created such a beautiful life for us through all of your deep spiritual work and self-care?" When my daughter expressed memories from her early childhood of my absenteeism (I was a workaholic until she was seven), and of a less-than-glowing review of how she recalls my role in dynamics with my family of origin, I felt devastated. I lost all sense of my own esteem because I had lost her approval in this high-stakes arena. She saw me as the villain in our story, and I had assumed I was the heroine.

The martyr's cry rang from my depths. *After all I've done for you? All the soul searching and courageous truth-telling and the road-paving and awakening and the dance parties and the organic food and, and, and!*

Here I was, a failure at, arguably, the most important and un-quittable job I'd ever have. I also saw that I had linked my success in mothering with much of my life's purpose, and here she was, robbing me of that importance.

The martyr has a hard time acknowledging that selflessness is an illusion. The truth is that I was never really doing any of it for her, because it's always for me. Offers that contain asks are wolves in sheep's clothing. Remember that one of the ways you can know that you were *always* doing it for yourself is your anger, resentment, or disappointment in someone who doesn't appreciate what you did for them. In this instance of ingratitude, the covert exchange was exposed, and the altruistic impulse revealed to be what it always was: need-meeting.

So, I wept and sobbed over her response (which she was merciful enough to text to me) in my bedroom alone that night and was able to really allow that part to experience the failure, embrace it, and own that part's belief that I was doomed to feel unseen, misunderstood, and rejected. And then, as the dust settled and the tears came to a pause, a voice rose up inside me: *Kelly, this is the reclamation opportunity! This is it, right here! Even if you've failed, you're also about to claim an experience of your own emotional courage and strength in service of yourself and your daughters.*

When I sat down with her to talk more about this, I was able to say those magic words: "Tell me more. I want to know more about your experience, more of what it was like." I sat with my daughter, and I listened to HER experience. I asked about her memories with authentic curiosity and reflected on how hard it must have been to have gone through what she did. I said, "I'm so sorry," as my eyes brimmed with heartfelt tears. I did not explain *my* side of the story, *my* why, nor the myriad defenses that had leapt to the mic to insist on the rightness and goodness of *my* choices. *I simply visited with hers.*

And of course, that defensive protector was present in the background, saying things like: *Well, but she needs to understand what really happened. She needs to know what it was like for me.* That part of me that needed to *get her to see.* And, because I have grown the capacity through titration and small practices of holding the sensation of my reality, I could allow all the parts inside to have their say while being present to what was actually in front of me: a precious human with whom my connection was more important than my rightness.

From there, I was able to empathize with what it was apparently like for her at that time, in a way I never would have imagined possible. And just beyond the roaring sensation of holding my own badness and wrongness, a new sensation rolled in like a luminescent fog. I felt pride. I knew this sensation, not from my 4.0s or book reviews, but because I'd been courageous like this before, and the formerly exiled part that now gets to remain in the room comes bearing gifts. This pride is the signature offering of my child self when she knows I've got her, and I am not leaving her side to enact the defenses that would otherwise shut her up and shut her feelings down.

Listening to my daughter at that moment made me remember that, as a kid, I didn't give a shit what my parents' story was. I didn't care why they were doing what they were doing. It couldn't have been less relevant to my experience. I was interested in *my* story and mine alone. Remembering this allowed me to anchor, to become more available to her experience, and to actually listen.

This was a profound opportunity for her to assess how safe I am as a parent, to experience how much room there is in this connection for her to have a different reality and specifically a different narrative about me, even one that does not frame me in the light that I prefer. After that point, from my experience, our relationship entirely changed. This experience birthed a new kind of affection, togetherness, openness and trust, all that came online somehow from my being characterized in this really shitty way.

And it was all made possible through my ability to wear the Villain Crown of the mother who did it wrong. Through this practice, I believe my daughter got the memo that it's not her job to tend to the part of me that is terrified of wearing that Villain Crown, and that it's not her job to manage my emotions, nor to maintain my self-concept.

These days I get Winter Solstice cards like this one (published with her permission!), and I know that I'm on the road to sovereign love.

> Dear Mama,   12/19/22
>
> Happy Solstice!!!
>
> In this past year, I have seen so much growth in you, and in us. You are blossoming, a pheonix from the ashes, into a brave, beautiful, strong, amazing woman that I already knew you to be. You are an embodiment of life. Wild, exciting, warm, fierce, all of it. You stand by me when you don't agree with me, when your angry or sad, you're still there. There are not moments where I doubt your love for me. Your ability to love so fully is one of the most magical parts of the blessing of having you as my mother in this life. Your listening to my problems, your advice, your jokes, your passions, and endless knowledge all amaze me. Keep being amazing ♡☉ —Sofia

135

The more you steep in the bittersweet practice of wearing the mothering edition of the Villain Crown, the more you witness true intimacy in your relationship with your children. This, I believe, is how true and lasting intimacy takes root. To support your process, here are two of my favorite modalities for gently exposing the inner dimensions that we bring to the table.

Parts Work and Family Constellations

PARTS WORK

You contain multitudes, and getting to know the different parts within is both vulnerable and beautiful. Parts work is essentially a way to be in dialogue with the different aspects of yourself in service of connecting to your own essential nature.

Dick Schwartz, founder of Internal Family Systems, wrote a book called *No Bad Parts* about, well. . . how there are no bad parts of you! The part that eats the extra cake, smokes the cigarette, signs up for yet another self-help program, or induces the panic attack are all protectors and managers here to serve the system. *They are all you—* just dimensions of you that have been fragmented away from your conscious awareness, arrested in stages of childhood. Our charged emotions, both positive and negative (including numbness), have a purpose. There are things that we get to say, to feel and not feel, to do and not do, because of the parts of us in charge of our protection.[1]

Your protector parts and so-called firefighter parts are all charged with keeping you from feeling the more painful emotions of shame, fear, loneliness, worthlessness, or powerlessness that are held by so-called exiles. Protectors keep you from triggering the tender feeling exiles, and firefighters are activated if the exiles have already been triggered, swooping in to put out the fire with dissociation, mania, addiction, or even suicidality. And until you let them know that their services are appreciated but no longer needed, these protectors work tirelessly, thanklessly *for* you to avoid deeper hurts.

Getting to know these parts of you is like introducing the members of a cast to one another in broad daylight after they've been performing in the dark (each one thinking that they were the star of a one-person show). But now these dimensions of yourself get to choose their assigned tasks, develop *intentional* relationships, and play together instead of carrying huge emotional burdens. It's up to you to genuinely learn about the stories these parts hold so as not to reject these aspects of yourself in judgment.

When I started engaging in parts work, I met a variety of different characters that have taken on various roles within my psyche. In one of my first parts work sessions with Tom Holmes, I was guided to meet the cast of characters around a dynamic I'd been experiencing. The first part I met was what I call "the cheerleader"—she was cheering me on, encouraging me to prepare for an encounter I had been worried about having. It was clear that this part had really gotten me through much of life. She's the one who always had the sassy response, aced the tests, perfected the performance—she's essentially the Type A driving force behind so many of my achievements in life. She loves preparation. As the session continued, I met the origin of the worry in a part that ran worst-case scenarios in front of my eyes like a news ticker tape, in an attempt to prepare me in her own way.

Shortly after meeting these two parts, Tom asked "How do you feel about these two parts working together?" From there, I immediately met a part who wanted to hunch over and hide away, emanating a judgy, critical, "better than you" energy that looked down on the previously assembled cast, as if to say, *what is wrong with you that you're this worried and freaked out and trying so hard? Play it cool, please.*

Tom helped me locate and track these various parts of my psyche, and their associated sensations in my body, as we watched their Broadway show. We tracked the dynamics back to an exile, whom all the aforementioned parts were charged with keeping, well *exiled*, so that the feelings held would not be felt. This exile presented as a child part that looked like a little girl in a business suit, holding buried feelings of pain, shame, sadness, and grief. She felt overly responsible for taking care of *everything* because of challenges she'd witnessed her mother experience, and it was almost as if she wanted to vomit up the burden. An incredibly striking realization occurred to me as I recognized a matrilineal imprint of this burden in women of my family that even manifested as vertigo and vomiting. Ultimately, we helped this part of me see there could be a world where she wasn't responsible for everything anymore, where she could unburden, and where *I*, as the Self, could offer her what she needed. Disburdened, she showed me what she'd rather be doing, which is playing with cats and prancing around in a tutu, so off she went!

Parts work can be a high yield way to connect and communicate with the dimensions of you that are crying out *"There's no other way for it to be than this!"* generating fluidity, flexibility, and compassionate shifts in perspective only possible with the capital S self has come online. The Self has what Schwartz refers to as the 8 Cs of Self Energy: compassion, curiosity, calm, confidence, creativity, clarity, courage, and connectedness. He writes: "The more you become familiar with it [the Self], the easier you can detect when you depart from that state—when you're having a 'part attack.' It stops becoming such a big deal, because you know it's temporary and that you can unblend from the part and help it out. . . . Many of our troubles come not so much from the part attack itself, but more from our panic about it, because we believe it defines us and won't end."[2]

He goes on to say, "When people spend time exploring inside, they all come to the same conclusion—that this essential Self is who we really are. I think that what's often called awakening or enlightenment is the embodied realization of that fact, and that shift from identifying with your parts and their burdens to identifying as your Self has profound implications."[3] As you'll discover by wading into the freeing modality of parts work, when your inner parts see each other and are relieved from the vigilance of protecting you from feeling past feelings, they offer gifts of imagination, creativity, and sweetness. Gifts that come with a sense of true expansion, true spaciousness, and delightful possibility.

SELF-LED PARTS WORK

Pick something that feels like a three out of ten on the emotional distress scale, and let's take some time to get curious about what it's trying to teach you. Remember, this isn't about fixing. Your protector feelings aren't the enemy, and they don't need to be defeated or vanquished. They are a necessary part of you and are there to serve you.

This is an eyes-closed, heart-open process, so get comfortable (pause and see if there's anything you need to be *juuuuusssstttt* a bit more comfy) and prepare yourself for expansion. Feel your spine, your feet, your points of contact with the chair and floor, notice your breath, and ground into safety in the present moment.

Choose a feeling that has come up for you more than once and think back not only to the last time it surfaced, but also the very first time you felt it. Try to fully conjure it and invite it to take center stage, just for a minute. Feel where it rests in your body.

139

Sometimes these feelings appear like big black bowling balls, or bright colorful light, or even prickling lightning bolts. Get curious about how they appear for you; the more you practice, the more intimacy you'll develop around their signs and signatures.

Breathe, and allow this facet of yourself to just be with you. Offer this part of you your love and compassion just by allowing it to be, without fixing or editing.

For myself, I'm thinking back to a time when something in my business didn't go quite as planned. I was disappointed, to say the least, and I often feel disappointment in my chest.

First there's a squeezing sensation, and sometimes, if the disappointment is profound, I'll feel the energy drop heavily into my upper belly.

When these facets of yourself show up, it's important to honor them and approach them with open-minded curiosity.

Ask non-judgmental questions like:

"What would happen if you didn't make sure I knew this feeling was important?"
"What would happen if you stopped doing your job of being right about how wronged I am?"
"What do I get because you exist? What do I get because of that? And because of that?"

. . . and so on.

In the case of my business disappointment, the answer is: I'd be taken advantage of, or I'd lose something that I'd then have to find somewhere else, putting me behind, and then I would feel less worthy. So, what I get is actually a feeling of fulfillment and worthiness. Well, that's a benevolent intent if I ever heard one!

Think back to the earliest times these sensations came online. What stories have you created around these feelings, and how have they served you over the years?

Honor where they first showed up, then welcome them to join you in the present, where you can hold space for them and give them what they need to feel resolved.

Ask yourself what those feelings might have wanted from you when you were younger?

Did she want to have her hair brushed?
Does she want to play with kitties?
Does she want a hug? Or to take a bath? Or just be still and sit with you?

Often feelings like disappointment are a surface mask for fear or longing, and compassionate empathy is the best treatment.

Figure out what those feelings are asking for, and lovingly offer it to them. This can be in your imagination, as you act out an exercise of safety and containment. It can also be physical, as you hug your body in order to let those feelings feel seen and loved.

> When you're done, thank these protector aspects for their vigilance and release them with gratitude and appreciation.
>
> In this way, you can allow those feelings to be a productive and supportive part of your own evolution, and through this seemingly simple exercise, you'll be able to embrace a dimension of yourself that is holding creative gifts while liberating your own protectors to use their energy for better things, like inspiring you and filling you with the joy of discovery.

FAMILY CONSTELLATIONS

It had been four years since I had sat down with my parents socially, after a rupture, the immensity of which I could never have foreseen. We had attended several sessions of family therapy, and then we retreated to our respective life corners with only superficial exchanges related to my children.

As a lifelong secular materialist, awakened into the cozy womb of the New Age, I have tried every modality that's crossed my path, with a sort of anthropological bemusement around what people study and do with themselves in order to somehow, someway, feel better. So, when my friend Dani suggested I try Family Constellations with Amerly Centeno, I was game!

Family Constellations is a therapeutic modality developed by Bert Hellinger in the 1990s that suggests that our personal struggles have roots in our family systems. The philosophy of *familienaufstellung* or "family positioning" posits that people unconsciously perceive patterns and structures within family relationships, which become schemas that influence their behavior. Amerly Centeno writes, "A family system is formed by energy, emotion, and information that connects all its members. Feelings, behaviors, and symptoms are not linked to one's personal history, but have their origins in 'family loyalty' to our ancestors."[4]

Hellinger refined what he called "The Orders of Love" as the basic governing forces of humans: inherited systems and hierarchies that often operate unconsciously in the collective consciousness, generated by family habits, beliefs, and practices. Centeno teaches that these Orders of Love can be broken down into three different subcategories: Belonging, Hierarchy, and the Balance Between Giving and Taking.

Belonging is a basic human need: the need to peacefully connect with a deep sense of being wanted, needed, and valued in the family group, larger community, and even place in society. Exclusion can have severe impacts on identity, self-esteem, recognition, and projection. Estranged family members, parental discord, and other alignments in a system can generate patterns that compensate for the rejection of a given person by others in the system. Even perpetrators and miscarried and aborted babies require acceptance into a system for the system to be ordered.

Hierarchy is often qualified by time, as in the order in which children are born, the timeline of when relationships are established, and the seniority of the person's role in the family, community, or really any social organization. Challenges in the hierarchy often manifest as parentified children who act as parents, siblings, or spouses to their own parents. The ordering of ancestors, parents, siblings, exes, and children must be established for a system's energy to flow.

When addressing the balance between Giving and Taking, it's important to remember that nothing happens in a vacuum. Every living thing takes something to survive, and knowingly or not, gives something back. Likewise, a family system requires constant give and take, but when the balance is skewed, the system breaks down. Taking the traditions and expectations of your family can be an effort to repay the balance of the life that they gave you, but there's only so much you can do to compensate before the giving is out of balance again. To give more than can be received and more than is given back becomes an act of disharmony rather than generosity.

The primary goal of constellations is to explore these transgenerational conflicts and *release* each family member from the heavy burdens of their ancestral history. For example, let's say your family's history contains a lot of domestic violence. If unaddressed, this issue presents an energetic imbalance, which can manifest generationally as a repeat pattern. In other words, you can expect to see the "apple doesn't fall far from the tree" situation playing out regularly in your family life. To "constellate" means that you're taking on your "rightful place" in your family line, resolving "loyalties" to past struggles that aren't yours to uphold.

On the day of the group family constellations event, eight of us took turns constellating. In each movement, we watched children parenting parents, grandfathers exiled, mothers burdened by miscarried babies, and husbands in hopeless death postures on the ground. Arranged by the constellator, the only prompt for the participants was "how do you feel?" Somehow, through forces unseen, these sometimes-strangers revealed behaviors and patterns that confronted the constellator like a forceful embrace. The kind of hug that says: *see, this is why it's felt this way.*

When it was my turn to constellate, I watched dynamics between my parents, my then husband, and my inner child play out with accuracy that left me speechless. With Amerly's sage guidance, healing phrases were spoken, and we were organized in proper alignment with my father behind me to my right, my mother behind me to my left, and my inner child in front of me. I went home that day and took a rare bath, perhaps because I thought that was what a woman who needed to take nurturing care of herself would do. As I rested into the warm water, I felt how important this day had been, and how irrelevant the mechanistic analysis truly was. Four days later, I reached out to my mom, invited her over for tea, and sat down with her for what felt like a human-sized interaction. A simple, down-to-earth, *hey, here's where I'm at* chat. I had set a two-hour container and checked in with myself every twenty minutes to ascertain that I was still a *Yes,*

143

and when we hugged goodbye, the next chapter of our relationship as mother and daughter began.

As you touch into your self-reclamation and intimately tend to the *Yes* and *No* inside, the fabric of your lifescape can't help but shift in morphic resonance. The people in your life who matter most to you will perceive and receive your energy differently, because you are forever changed, giving them space to show up differently in turn. There will be manifestations that spring from your newfound magnetism, more so with shadow alchemy than with any so-called positive thinking.

BALANCE YOUR INNER KING & QUEEN

Also adapted from Amerly, this visualization will help you internalize and reconcile your family constellation.

Take a deep breath. In this visualization, you're the trunk of your family tree. *Be* the trunk.

Imagine your birth parents as a big split in your trunk, two main branches that diverge, to form their own forked junctions with their own parents, and their parents' parents. If someone replaced your mother or father, or their mothers or fathers, add a branch coming off their junction.

Add another branch for every sibling, teacher, and friend who has touched, informed, or changed them, until there's a whole society and culture of branches entangled and entwined with supports, debts, and life weight.

Internally turn to look at them, the many generations and even strangers who have entangled with family members through debts, violations, or persecution.

Look back and acknowledge how all the parts shaped your trunk, and internally, say *Thank You* to all the branches that have gathered sun and rain to nourish you, and the roots that draw up the essence of life to enrich you.

Look at your life, and really *see* it, in its entirety, and see its part in existence as a whole.

Look at your life and say YES!

CHAPTER 10

Sexual Shame Alchemy

All my life, I've judged flirty girls. Solicitous, suggestive, and sexually provocative women, in dress or behavior, used to really rub me wrong. All the while, I went through an extensive phase where I had primarily male friends, leveraging my sexual energy covertly so that I could plausibly deny that I was baiting any of them into believing that I might someday, somehow, be available.

That's probably why, on a semi-conscious level, I knew that the path home to myself would require that I walk intentionally and consciously toward this energy field. Luckily, I manifested some amazing women to neutralize my rejection through the pleasure of their presence (I honored them in a collection I offer called Faces of Fierce Femininity and in my in-person event, Audacious Embodiment), and I began to try on, literally and figuratively, booty shorts, hooker boots, twerking, pole, and flirting. After years in a relationship where I shut down my sexual energy outside of the bedroom to seal a monogamous container, it took some serious audacity to imagine that I had permission to explore the seductress archetype, to run my non-genital sexual energy, to play out in the world, and to begin to open these channels for *myself.*

Several years into ending my second marriage and exploring intentional celibacy, I can tell you that sexual energy isn't what we've been led to believe. It's imaginal energy, creative energy, and our very life force. In fact, since I haven't been having sex, I've created, created, and created some more. I've learned to dance, sing, sew, decorate, put on live events, podcast, and mother with laughter and play. I softened, I lightened up, and I integrated more and more life from the places where fear and shame had taken up residence in my body.

But it wasn't all gumdrops and roses. During this time, I walked over the fiery coals of admonition from other women for sharing dance videos and strutting far outside the lines of my prescribed (no pun intended) professional lane. I lost a hundred thousand newsletter subscribers (almost half of the tribe I'd collected), and after about a year of entering through the upset with each and every incident of triggering rejection, I felt the tsunami of this initiation to a more plastic identity finally receding.

Perhaps I was *now* a sexually liberated and integrated woman!

I decided that a new challenge for me would be to practice receiving, and I chose to open rather than close when (perhaps unwanted) male attention was directed my way. I would walk open and smiling, say thank you, and watch with love the part of me that imagines there are always strings attached to every offering.

So, when I got pulled over for going a few miles over the speed limit, I felt an opportunity. I could have gone all sovereign and declared my rights as a living woman. I could have denied or fought. I could have gone dark witch. But I decided, *I'm gonna play with this*, when a super handsome cop I'd seen a hundred times approached my window. He introduced himself and his role and I replied with coyness, "Oh I knowwww . . . .I notice you every day." Well, I didn't get a ticket that day, and it was simply a light energetic exchange. About twenty minutes later, I was driving under some Miami old growth trees, and a huge branch turned my windshield into a mosaic in seconds. I don't believe in accidents. I believe that we attract these "random" events when it serves us to do so; an accident is a marvelous way to secure punishment while remaining innocent. Is it possible that I felt the need to be punished for expressing my sexual energy so overtly, for flirting outright? When that expression is met with punishment, I'm suddenly in a space that feels familiar, and, ironically safer, and maybe even enjoyable because I don't get to celebrate (which comes with all sorts of risks); I get to complain!

I recognized this pattern from the early days of my pole journey when I injured my ribs doing a relatively basic move, not once, but three times.

So, what might my belief be?

That irresponsibly sexual women get punished.

Those women are bad.

If I become (a version) of those women, I get punished.

The world makes sense.

Alchemizing sexual shame and fear requires that we walk through the portal of our judgments home to a deeper understanding of eros as a birthright entitlement in this human body. Learning how to own, wield, and master sexual energy may be one of the most important spiritual commitments we can choose to make. But how do we make such a commitment in a climate that has split the Madonna from the whore? Where tantric light and love-energetic spiritual sex is better than carnal, buttons-flying, hair-pulling sex? Where hookup culture has us judging puritans and puritans judging one-night-standers?

Sex and sexuality are a reclamation so personal that even endeavoring to write this chapter is probably somewhat misguided. I know, however, that there are some important questions to ask, and so I'll share what I think they might be:

What are your sex rules?

Which ones did you inherit, and which are learned from personal experience?

How is sex allowed and not allowed in your life and in the lives of others?

How do you feel judged by others in society for your choices around sex and sexuality?

How do you judge others for theirs?

What would make your relationship with sex and sexuality healthier?

Maybe you've decided that you can't live without sex, you're entitled to impose your sexual energy on everyone everywhere, and sex is the same as breathing. You feel pity for the repressed, tight, under-fucked women who cast aspersions your way. Or maybe you're on the side of what's pure and sacred, and you feel that sexual energy belongs in the marital suite and nowhere else. You see breaches beyond the bedroom as a core rot in society, and you're pretty damn sure that women flaunting anything are lost at best and liabilities at worst.

Wherever you are on the archetypal spectrum, if you're triggered about sexuality, yours or someone else's, you're split inside, just like me. There's a part of you that is righteously protecting your personal status quo and a part that wants to know: yeah, but if I was *that* other way, would I still be lovable? These inner tensions are where struggles and patterns of suffering arise, and they represent an always-front-row seat to exactly that which you reject, whatever it may be. It's right in your face. This war is fueled by shame that keeps the less-identified part under wraps and also drives addictions through the energizing of the taboo.

149

Shame is a social management emotion; when it comes up, it's meant to organize and redirect your behavior to line up with what you believe makes you a good girl or bad girl. Shame inherently feels like it *shouldn't* be there. When shame comes up for me, it feels like a deep heat emanating from the core of my being that tracks all the way up my throat and my head and under my arms. This somatic sequence is the most powerful warning that can be issued from my inner protectors and it says, *figure out any way to be right immediately.* As a result, you likely do everything in your power to smother the parts of you that can spark sensations of shame. But shame cannot exist where there is honest acknowledgement and curiosity. If you can grow the capacity to expose your shame to the light of your awareness and simply *be* with it, you will meet the parts of yourself that shame is protecting, and you will see how sweet, innocent, and wide-eyed they are.

RECLAMATION REMEDY:
ALCHEMIZE SHAME IN YOUR BODY

I learned this exercise from my girl, Daniela Garcia, a.k.a. The Joy Alchemist, and it *will* help you alchemize your shame.

1. Adorn an eye mask or blindfold so you can disconnect from how you *see* your body, and instead connect with how you *feel* in the parts of your body that you aren't into or tend to critique. Spend five to ten minutes connecting with those parts, listening to your own inner critic.

2. Now, remove your eye mask. Stand in front of a full-length mirror and spend another five to ten minutes reconnecting with your inner judge, only this time with your eyes wide open, looking directly at the parts of your body you're being so harsh about.

3. Now, get comfy, because this is going to feel a bit uncomfortable. Close your eyes and send your gaze inwards again—don't shy away from the feeling, sensations, and emotions that have come up as you openly sit in judgment of yourself. This aspect is a part of you, and you need to connect with it, give it permission to exist, and allow it to express through you.

4. Shake it off. Like, literally get up and shake all those thoughts and feelings through your body. Play some music, dance it out, and liberate all the heavy body shame into feelings of acceptance and forgiveness.

5. Find the safe space you created in front of the mirror and give your body a voice. Speak as if you were those parts and say all the things you think it would feel in response to your shame and judgment. For example, your belly. "I turn the fuel

you eat into energy, and I hold your intuition, but I always feel like you wish I was something different. You suck me in, you cover me up, you never make me loved or valued. I wish I wasn't something you hated so much you wish others couldn't see me." Or your thighs: "I carry you throughout your day and help you climb every obstacle in your way, but you call me Thunder Thighs and poke at my dimples like they aren't adorable. I'd love to feel the breeze sometime, but you're too ashamed of me to wear skirts or shorts. I wish you could see my strength instead of wanting me to be smaller."

6. While remaining cozy, give those places you've been hating on some love. You could massage them, squeeze them, or just touch them and say, "Thank you!" Let those parts receive your love and gratitude for ten minutes. You can dance, bend, and stretch, or even rub scented oils as you celebrate the parts of you that you usually vilify.

151

Take a few minutes to come down from this exercise. It can be difficult to transmute ingrained feelings of shame and disdain, so refresh and reorient by doing some gentle breathing, sending the breath to all the parts of your body, allowing a sense of wholeness to come over you as you reconcile all the beautiful parts of you.[1]

Shame to Pride Posture
In this exercise, we want to call up a feeling of shame we have over one of our more villainous shadow traits. (For reference, I did this practice recently when my friend told me that I had a nasty habit of telling her how *she* feels. And I knew she was right.)

Call up the sensation of being pinned by shame, a sense of inescapable culpability, wrongness, and badness. Notice where it sits in your body, and what your body *wants to do*. Often, there's an urge to look away from the inconvenient truth, so you turn your head and cast your eyes downwards. Sometimes there's a tightness in your chest or throat, or a sinking feeling in your stomach, so you hunch forward to protect those areas.

In this exercise, I want you to lean into those gestures, and relax into that posture.

Avert your gaze. Like a marionette whose strings have been cut, allow your head to drop down as you sink into your ribcage.

Rest there for a bit. Allow your body to feel that protection and aversion.

When you're ready, reverse the motion. Open your eyes and direct your gaze with honesty and pride. Raise your head, and draw in a big breath, inflating your chest and pulling your shoulders back as your spine straightens and lengthens, vertebrae by vertebrae.

Notice that this feels like the opposite of shamefully hiding your villain side. Instead, embrace the antidote to shame and become proud of the qualities you tried to deny.

Repeat these posture changes, super slowly, a few times, and notice how it feels when you come out of your shameful hunch.

Allow the somatic sense memory of shame from your childhood to connect to its native antidote. Expand your range and release what's stored, often from decades prior, and wants to move.[2]

What if a camera crew were following you?
It's time to turn your life into your very own episode of *The Office*, complete with side-eye camera angles and even a B Reel of hot-take commentary.

> Pretend you're being followed around by a camera crew, and look back over your day and be honest about the behaviors you wouldn't want in the final edit.
>
> What can you own in your daily experience that you wouldn't necessarily want broadcasted for your boss, your mom, or even your homeowners' association to see? Are you scarfing your less-than-Instagrammable lunch while scrolling? Is your room a disaster zone? Did you snap at your son in a way you wouldn't be caught dead speaking to a friend?
>
> Get familiar with the behaviors you engage in daily that you're potentially ashamed of, and know that you can't hide from you. How might you refine, optimize, or adjust said behaviors so that you can move through your life with more integrity and less inner tension? Not for anyone's gaze, but for your own coherence.

In Western society, sex is painted as wildly taboo. We don't really talk about what turns us on, since it's deemed shameful to talk about the dirty, dark fantasies that lie dormant and unattended in our psyches. You likely grew up being motivated towards "abstinence," taught about all the *negative* associations with sex: pregnancy, STDs, and heartless men. In essence, you've been made to feel like your sexuality is a problem, practically right out of the gate.

As my dear friend and absolute queen in the realm of conscious kink, Kimi Inch, put it when I interviewed her on my podcast: "Sexual shame comes from a lack of permission for yourself and your partners. Is there a way that we can make friends with our shame and embrace it? So that it's not standing in our way, but it's actually catapulting us into a deeper sense of intensity and excitement during our interactions with our partners."[3]

As humans, our nervous systems have developed to hold a wide array of intense emotions, including shame, and often what's needed is the permission to orient toward the sensations and allow them residence. When we *turn towards* that intensity, we find that release, relief, and expansion are mere moments away. Somehow, the courage to hold shame is rewarded with pleasure. I've found that the most powerful toolkit for ritualized sexual shame alchemy lies in the world of conscious kink and BDSM (Bondage/Discipline, Dominance/ Submission, and Sadism/Masochism).

BDSM: The Unlikely Therapeutic

As humans, we've got a lot of different kinks. Voyeurism, exhibitionism, sexual masochism or sadism, fetishism . . . and exploring these portals of arousal can lead to ecstatic reclamation. But when these proclivities are cloaked in shame, they are distorted into furtive addictions, self-recrimination, and even sociopathic mistreatment of others.

As my BDSM teacher Om Rupani writes in his book *Prerequisites to Ecstasy*, "We all have a visceral understanding of what NONCONSENSUAL domination and submission is. Every headline in every newspaper on every single day is pretty much a story of nonconsensual domination and submission . . . Consensual domination and submission is anchored in two people giving each other what they truly want."[4]

We are familiar with power dynamics. We've been harmed by them and naturally fear them, but is it possible that we are also aroused by them? Of course it is! Because our traumas are eroticized, beckoning us home through fantasy, so that we can claim the *Yes* underneath the *No*. I've sometimes mused that the closest most people get to engaging in kink power play is a visit to the doctor where they get to be dominated by someone who accesses their body, tells them what to do, and punishes them for disobedience. Hopefully what a doctor visit and BDSM do have in common is consent.

In BDSM culture, consent and communication around safe and explicit checklists of yes's and no's and everything in between are approached in advance of play. Amazingly, most couples don't discuss sex, what works for them, what doesn't, what they want and don't want, unless there's a problem. It's the *this-seems-to-be-going-fine-let's-hope-for-the-best-hope-he-can-read-my-mind* approach. In contrast, proactive, explicit, and clear communication is a prerequisite for couples engaging in BDSM. And once you get good at expressing needs and boundaries in the bedroom, this skill serves you in the reality of your everyday life as well.

In BDSM, the Submissive (who may appear as the "victim") sets the parameters for her own sensory stimulation; these parameters often involve impact play, bondage, and other approaches to "coming into her body" so that she can fully surrender control in the safe conditions of a bigger energy handling her *for* her pleasure and embodied experience. The Dom, on the other hand, experiences his own divine power, creating the conditions for his Sub to move into liminal spaces only possible because of his mastery. She is attuned inward and he is attuned outward while also feeling his own system. Sub/Dom (or "follower/leader") practices can offer anyone who has suffered some form of sexual abuse the chance to alchemize shame and rewrite a narrative that has been engrained as a deep trauma in the soma. For example, you get to electively eroticize an experience of abuse, bringing a *Yes* where there is only *No* in the body, *or* you can rewrite history and play out a scene where you tell your abuser: "Fuck you, get off me!" You can finally heal that shame about your breasts, or playfully craft scenes to dramatize your jealousy rather than nitpick and criticize your man's behavior. Release, expansion, and ecstatic states can be accessed through the gates of taboo between consenting adults.

And like partner dancing, power dynamics and organized roles don't need to be sexual to be alchemically powerful. During my in-person event, Audacious Embodiment, Kimi Inch demo'ed a spanking session on me in front of a hundred women, where she lovingly struck me for all of the times I doubted and belittled myself. She acted as my higher self "punishing" me back into my aligned expression. I was anchored in my body because of the impact sensation and the grief that lived underneath my self-betrayal moved out through my tears, as it seemed to for every woman in the room. It was nothing short of game-changing for me in a way that talk therapy never could be. I've come to believe that the creativity and imagination that is brought to otherwise fixed dimensions of shame is, itself, a part of the healing.

CAN BDSM HEAL THE WORLD?
The Healing Properties of BDSM

Improved communication and boundaries

When you become practiced at learning your *No's*, using safe words, and identifying what really gets you off, you bring this kind of self-awareness to the rest of your life and to the world. Long gone are the days of hoping and praying that someone will read your mind and then experiencing delicious resentment when they fail to do so. BDSM affirms that it's your job to be clear about creating the conditions for safety and fulfillment of needs in your lifescape, and it's your responsibility to treat yourself with the care, nurturance, and respect that a good Dom would.

Ultimately, clearer *Yes*'s and clearer *No*'s lead to more secure attachment and emergent trust. In fact, the results of a research survey of 902 BDSM and 434 control participants conducted by psychologist Andreas Wismeijer indicated that "people in the BDSM scene reported higher levels of wellbeing in the past two weeks than people outside it, and they reported more secure feelings of attachment in their relationships."[5]

Get high and experience inner peace

Interestingly, pain and impact play during BDSM can have a calming and meditative effect. Many Submissives describe pain play (where they control the intensity) as one of the only means to effectively quiet their minds. When individuals are experiencing intense pain, their minds may become focused on the sensation of pain itself, and a complex inner pharmacopeia of endorphins seem to lace in and out of what would otherwise be unwanted sensations. This can create a sense of mindfulness or meditation, as the individual becomes fully immersed in the present moment and their immediate physical experience, taking them out of their heads and into their bodies.

A handful of scientific studies have found that BDSM interactions can create brain activity changes that are associated with pleasure[6] as well as measurable alterations in neuromodulatory molecules such as oxytocin, beta-endorphins, and endocannabinoids.[7] These changes in brain blood flow and chemical messengers have been documented as being a meditation or "yoga-like" benefit for the Submissive,[8] as well as a "flow state" benefit for the Dom.[9] Preliminary research suggests endocrine parameters that correlate with the observed and experienced phenomena of flow, creation and connection, and self-enhancement.[10]

Increased intimacy

When you invest in complementarity with a partner, when you show them the whole you (including your shame and vulnerable points), when you entrust them or are entrusted, intimacy is inevitable. BDSM offers a framework to resolve the all-too-common pathology of cowering, insecure men and hen-pecking controlling women; when we get into Dom/Sub dynamics, a safety and coherence returns to the field that creates the conditions for true connection. Nowadays, studies are finding that couples who participate in these practices have decreased levels of physiological stress and increased relationship closeness.[11]

Access to wellbeing

For true wellness and self-love, there is no avoiding the essential reclamation that is our sexuality, which is enmeshed with our sense of worth, lovability, pleasure, trust, and even access to our own divine nature. Especially for those with sexual trauma—and let's be honest; all of us have some form of trauma around sex—BDSM can help transform and transmute the confusion that is locked up in one's relationship to their own sexuality.[12] I believe that the role that sexuality plays in our lives is a Gordian knot aching to be released.

And in a holofractal universe, as we relax and release our fear-based habits and step into our true power, through domination or submission, we reclaim vital force energy that melts illness and dis-ease. This vital force energy—eros—radiates outward into all our relationships and actions, creating an impact too beautiful to be measured.

BDSM and conscious kink can offer practices that create the conditions for the reclamation and journey back to yourself. And wouldn't it be funny if this intentional exploration has been so maligned and pathologized because of its power? A power that all of us can access as we relax into the alchemical container of the age-old technology of adult, consensual, erotic relationship. The system would love to remain in charge of determining who's been a bad girl, who hasn't, and who gets what punishment, but wouldn't it be better to empower your man to do that for you?

The Maturation of Your No

By this point, you're likely developing a deeper kind of intimacy with your precious *No*, both outside and inside yourself. The *No* is the pattern disrupt you need to awaken true, conscious, meaningful change, and sometimes this relational journey begins with a huge *No* (let's be real: a *Fuck No!*), which means standing up for your truth even when a part of you is terrified you might suffer permanent consequences for doing so. This initiation is a courageous act of self-advocacy. I've learned that when you are willing to embrace your inner dark witch, Kali, Medusa, or dominatrix you are reclaiming the "don't fuck with me" style woman within you who is able to hold onto her *No* ferociously in the name of a greater, deeper experience of love.

Kimi Inch says that boundaries can be about inviting more pleasure into your life, rather than aversive self-protection. When you say "no," you're simultaneously saying "yes" to something you imagine will feel better. Setting an empowered boundary is not just about claiming your *No* (which can keep you stuck in the close walls of rigidity); it's about opening your arms to more appreciation and alignment in your choices, all in the most loving and nurturing way possible.

The early stages of your masculine reclamation have rigid boundaries, rigid *No*'s; you might cut people out of your life or develop a staunch meditation practice. Having a hard boundary helps you advocate for yourself and turn down the noise. Revisiting our story, this is how the miller who took the poor bargain can *become* the king who will fully love up and devote to his maiden, so she can come into the full flower of her feminine.

The mature masculine decision-maker doesn't follow a rule book and punish deviations, however. He assesses each and every moment, attunes to the feminine, and makes wise choices based on what is needed. For example, during my Reclaimed Woman era of the last several years, I moved beyond rigid dietary rules, embracing a sovereign relationship with food based on loving preferences after fifteen years of staunch rigidity. I distinctly remember a day that I checked in with my gut, and the memo I got was *Go buy Breyers ice cream!* (a staple of my tween years). I completely rejected the message, insisting that I needed to be *more* rigid with my diet instead of *less*. Days later, I found two Entenmann's donuts—the literal emblem of pleasure from my late childhood—wrapped in a napkin on the floor of my daughter's room. Before my health reclamation, I would eat an entire box of chocolate-covered donuts dipped in my coffee, and I'm not sure anything could have been better than that. But after several decades,

159

these donuts mysteriously showed up in my house just days after I'd resisted the taunting suggestion of Breyers ice cream from my inner recesses, and I could feel the cosmic wink in this opportunity.

I'd been holding onto a rigidity and dogmatism that had served me and now was overstaying his welcome, arresting me in an immature state of my inner masculine. Thus, my feminine was arrested as well; my relationship to my impulses, my desires, and my pleasures are all aspects of my own inner little girl who is longing for these taboo foods that are holding all this vital force energy.

I made a small ritual out of eating those donuts, dipping them in my chai latte and really being present with every bite. Afterward, I ick-ed at the filmy feeling in my mouth that I'd somehow selectively forgotten attended this processed food delight. In fact, my daughter said someone gave them to her and she wouldn't even eat them because they're "gross." And it was true; they were delicious, and they were gross! The donut eating was a needed jailbreak from the virtuousness of clean eating. It became as though taboo foods are in a glass cabinet clearly marked, *Thou Shalt Not Touch These*, and in some dimension of myself, I remained in devotion to them. In softening the rigid, reflexive, firm *No* boundaries and realizing that my intuition and impulses hold very valuable information and directions, I've proven to myself that I'm actually more resilient than formerly imagined.

So, the day will come when you can try the gluten again, see the sister again, do the unhealthy or unspiritual thing and still feel safe. If you remain in the rejection energy for too long, your self-sourced trust begins to erode, and the good/bad split is crystallized within. We become tight and judgmental, and others may experience our boundaries as a big, outstretched palm pushing life away.

Holding paradox is a hallmark of adult psychology. If feminism can be both an engineered psyop and a necessary stage of our actualization, if Top 40 hip hop can be both the result of MK-Ultra-entrained illuminati and also bring me experiences of tear-inducing delight when I dance, and if gluten can be poison and perhaps a delicious treat, then I can see with sobriety and choose without rejection of that which I am denying. I reclaim neuroception, and I avoid needing to source safety from rules. Instead, I trust. I trust my spine, my discernment, and my decision-making, and I also trust God, my path, and my process. If we allow it, our journeys will always lead us home to reconciling what Jung referred to as the *tension of opposites.*

Once you can make a sacred union of your inner polarities, you'll be able to say *Yes!* with absolute certainty that all parts of you are invited to the party, and *No!* when you know that not all aspects are on board. All these flavors and facets of your being, along with your personal pleasure protocol, set the tone for our play in Part 3.

PART 3
YES

CHAPTER 11

Feminine Homecoming

When the devil mixed the messages, the Handless Maiden felt that she had only one choice in order to survive: to return to the forest with her baby son. Two deer were sacrificed, their eyes and tongues saved as false evidence of mother and child's departure from this world. With tear-stained faces, the queen and the new mother bid each other farewell, and with the nursing infant nestled into her chest, the Handless Maiden was once again cast into the cold, dark night. Feeling raw, tender, tested, yet irrepressibly devoted to her journey, she left behind the beautiful life and all its trappings to venture back into the dark, untamed wilds of the woods.

She was not alone and adrift, however. Her heart filled with a familiar feeling of love and belonging as she reconnected with the spirit of the forest, who appeared by her side once again. Following the spirit's radiant glow, she eventually came upon a clearing. Wood smoke billowed up into the sky from a small cottage in a meadow.

The maiden approached the cottage, her babe still swaddled softly to her chest, and the door opened. A warm light spilled over the threshold amidst life-enhancing sounds of buoyant laughter, and a lively group of women, young and old, poured out to greet her. The maiden and son felt the embrace of true kinship as they were welcomed with open arms. Even in this forested place, far away from the king she loved so dearly, the maiden felt her spirits lift. She sighed out the stress and tension she had been holding in her heart, releasing dead air that had been stuck in her lungs.

As women of the woods (who knew the ancient, untold, wordless mysteries), this sublime coterie could see her for who she truly was. She delighted in the realization that she'd found a supportive sanctuary where she would be able to meet more of the dimensions hidden within her, due to the literal and existential exhale that women offer each other in sisterhood.

To be continued . . .

Back to the Forest Again

Nobody wants to go back into the darkness of the proverbial woods. But, since you've been doing your shadow work, owning your rejected and projected parts, maturing your inner masculine, and shedding beliefs, roles, and habits, you understand that this is about the journey, not the destination. The devil is still bound to show up to mix the messages, call your beautiful baby an actual dog, and expose all the ways you might still be taking the bait of fear and self-betrayal. In those confronting invitations back into the woods (your shadow), you will perceive the choice to fall into old patterns . . . *or* to put on your badass Reclaimed Woman boots as you hold your innocent child heart-close and remember that you *can* walk in the dark. In fact, as a woman, you were born to do just that.

As we explored in Part 2, shadow work is not for the faint of heart. By now you've taken your initiatory invitation, stopped trying to buy eggs from the hardware store, practiced entering through the upset, resolved superiority, and worn in your jewel-encrusted Villain Crown. You've likely found that drama, conflict, and complaint are beginning to quiet, and plot twists you couldn't have written are winding their way into your lifescape. Shadow work comes with rewards (*claiming the gems from your cave*) and gets easier as our inner safety resources shore up. And thank goodness it does, because there's no going back. There's no way to un-know, un-see, and un-do, and there's no crawling back up into the womb of rebirth.

The maiden cannot go back to who she was before the poor bargain or losing her hands. Nor can she forget the great love she now has, the king who relishes her wildness and her sweetness, who represents the love we can gift to ourselves. And, in the midst of your expansions, you too may find that the "devil" (a.k.a. your psyche's internal predator) returns to make sure you're still a hard *No* for self-abandonment.[1] It is a matter of soul life or death, after all, and feminine gifts must be delivered to ready arms. In his lovely interpretation and retelling of the "Handless Maiden," literary and mythic scholar Dr. Martin Shaw expresses that the woods are *"Never quite the same twice,"* somehow familiar and new every time.[2]

My own journey into discovering my *Yes* has taken me in some very humbling directions and raised more than a few eyebrows along the way, including my own. But behind every initial cringe, behind the confusion, behind the *wait-no!-seriously?!* was my inner child, peeking out from behind the curtain, wondering if she could come out in her tutu, carrying her magic wand with kitties and chickies in tow, to *finally* join the party. And it was always worth it. Every tight squeeze, dark night, and immolation of my life script rendered more of me available to me, giving me more of a sense of being in my own skin with less and less to hide and more and more to laugh about, marked by the delight of *it had to be just this way, didn't it?*

Central to Estés's interpretation of the tale is the idea that this story recounts the full spectrum of a woman's life in seven-year phases (all the way from birth to 105+); this is a story rooted in the theme of endurance. The maiden has summoned her inner masculine presence and attention—she's been seen, kissed, and loved by her king—but this time, she's delivered to the forest by her feminine, her queen, to *fully* become herself. She trusts her process: "The maiden is on her way again, wandering toward a great woods in all great faith that something will come from that great hall of trees, something soul-making."[3]

The woods shower her with grace.

Once again, the maiden meets her spirit guide, which we can see as the wise woman's spiritual center: her deeply felt intuition, her

167

inner feminine Godspark. Estés describes the guide as "the infinitely merciful nature of the deep psyche during a woman's journey. . . . This spirit who leads and shelters her is of the old Wild Mother, and as such is the instinctual psyche that always knows what comes next and what comes next after that."[4]

Because she is now strong in her Self, she can easily hear the whisper of her intuition, follow her inner *Yes* and *No,* and find her way to a cottage in a beautiful meadow, full of women ready to raise her up. That's right, woman! Your *Yes* gets to be so deliciously supported now that you've owned your *No,* and you will find your women, ready and waiting to love you. The stone always rises to meet the audacious footstep.

On the thrill of this female community, Shaw writes, "The glimpse of the women in the cottage will always walk with me, the rest of my life. . . . This does an end to the exhausted notion that every trial must always be faced alone. . . . She's done the hard yards and has encountered a whole cadre of women who have done the same, that gather her in, that warm her, that adore what she has brought into the world—her baby son."[5] These women too have taken the self-initiation journey and are here with hands on her back and so much love. It's not the final showdown of the hero's journey; as Shaw points out, there's no need to slay dragons. It's kinder and softer. It's a homecoming.

When we awaken to ourselves, our soul family hears that call and they come. These angelic friendships, romantic dynamics, and collaborative partnerships emerge from the fabric of your new life experience. The number of women who have seemingly fallen from the sky in the past few years of my journey assures me of the abundance that always awaits my receptivity. But I've only been able to enjoy this fabric of feminine containment and inspiration because I've learned to trust my impulses, each and every weird, irrational, and wild one of them, and they've led me to the connections that I've needed to grow.

Reclaim Your Biological Impulses

For many of us, our childhood impulses were synonymous with "bad behavior" and met with punitive, oppressive, and commandeering energy. *Ritalin anyone?* But now, as an adult, you're ready to honor your impulses, seeing them as your Godspark, and to trust that they are calling you back home.

One of the easiest ways to send your body the signal that you're here and that you care is to start with biology. Your body has wants and needs: warmth, food, water, sunlight, rest, and quiet. What if you listened like an attentive lover to her every little request? It might just be the start of a beautiful relationship. A shift both simple and profound, honoring your biological impulses looks like prioritizing what is wanted, whether it is a sweater or socks, water, picking up or putting down the fork. Start to listen, care, and respond in an attuned way, and feel the trust with your body build. Of all the biological impulses, my favorite, most game-changing practice has been to pee differently. I call it urinary reclamation.

When we, as women, choose to devote a little more time, care, and attention to peeing, it's a pattern disrupt of epic proportions. Honoring your biology in this way defies decades of conditioning that says: *What your body wants is less important than what is wanted from your body.*

Let that sink in.

I can't count the infinite times I've made my body wait until it was socially convenient to pee, the number of times I've promised to "pee quick" or to "be right back" and how often (when I believed in germ theory) peeing was just a way to rid myself of my partner's bacteria so as not to have future problems peeing. Amazingly, you can make a devotional practice out of honoring the impulse to pee when it arises, and to attend to the present and available pleasure in doing so.

There are 3 simple steps to this urinary reclamation practice:

1. Notice when you have the impulse to pee, and stop what you're doing.
2. If you are with others, do not imply that you will rush to maintain social connection or to minimize another's inconvenience while tending to your own needs. Banish, "I'm going to pee quick," "I'll be right back," and "I'll just be a minute" from your lexicon. Instead, you can say, "I need to use the bathroom," get up, go, and take your sweet time.
3. Bring your full attention to the sensory contrast as you move from the discomfort of having to pee to the pleasure of peeing and the relief of an empty bladder.

In this experience, you are attuning to your own impulses as they arise, starting with the most basic biological need of all. Once you prioritize honoring your biological impulses, you'll be available to bring awareness to creative ones. These impulses will drop in or rise up out of the void; they aren't products of decisions, contemplation, or consideration. You'll see a billboard and feel that you want to take salsa lessons, touch a shirt at a store and find yourself interested in operating a sewing machine, or bite into a carrot and feel a longing to grow your own. Wherever that flicker of *Yes* sparks, there is a watchful, serious, invested, and interested container protecting her from the wind. That doesn't mean you have to buy dancing shoes or all the seeds at the garden store, but it does mean you're going to take each impulse with devotional seriousness into your heart and make some space for it. I, personally, honor all my impulses because I know they lead me to grand adventures.

As I mentioned, when I moved to Miami in 2018, even though it was ostensibly for love, it was also for my body. It was the first time I was willing to actually listen to what my body wanted and needed—warmth and humidity—and what unfurled since that time is, well, the subject of this book! I showed up and served my body's desires, and she exhaled with gratitude. Every day that I wake up in this paradise and my muscles are warm, my skin dewy, and my dress gently blowing with a breeze that feels like nature making love to me, I smile at the leap I took, for myself and my feminine homecoming. Whether the moves your *Yes* engender are tiny or titanic in proportion, honoring your impulses and devoting yourself to yourself will start to alter the fabric of your lifescape, rather immediately, and often to surprising delight.

Estés describes the wild intensity of cravings thusly:

And then there are the cravings. Oh, la! A woman may crave to be near water, or be belly down, her face in the earth, smelling that wild smell . . . She may have to plant something, weed something, pull things out of the ground, or put them into the ground. She may have to knead and bake, rapt in dough up to her elbows . . . She may feel she will die if she does not dance naked in a thunderstorm, sit in perfect silence, return home ink-stained, paint-stained, tear-stained, moon-stained. A new self is on the way. Our inner lives, as we have known them, are about to change.[6]

These impulses are the language of desire, your mother tongue, and the reclamation of desire is where our *Yes* journey begins.

RECLAMATION REMEDY: WHAT DOES THE LITTLE GIRL INSIDE YOU WANT TO DO?

Women today experience one of two general problems; they're either completely overwhelmed and frazzled, or they feel totally numb. I like to think of overwhelm as the immature feminine, and numbness as the immature masculine, and the cheat code to maturing these energies is to learn how to get back into your body—*fast*.

It turns out the roads back in were paved early in life: song, dance, play, pleasure, and making things with our beautiful hands. Here's an exercise to help you reconnect with the little girl inside you when you feel like a stranger in your own skin. She knows what you need:

1. **Breathe.** Deeply but gently, without urgency, follow your breath in and out as you begin to relax.
2. **Visualize a safe space that brings you pleasure,** like a beach, a calm forest, a relaxing cabin, or even just your backyard. You want to feel like you're okay wherever you are, and nothing can harm or frighten you or your inner child.
3. Once you have that place in your mind, **invite your little girl to join you**, bringing all the innocence and vulnerability inherent to that young age. Connect to her through touch, eye contact, and presence.
4. **Ask her what would make her feel good, happy, and excited.** Listen to what she says, without judgment or direction.

Thank your inner girl for her guidance, and for letting you know what to prioritize in order to feel connected to her and to your body. Her needs won't always be the same, and each inquiry will offer direction in your healing journey.

CHAPTER 12

Reclaim Your Desire

As a woman, your desires are beautiful, righteous, and essential for the world to thrive. Enjoy the desires you have . . . Just love what you love, and want what you want without caveats . . . Women want anything and everything from wild, intimate sex, and delicious, healthy foods, to great clothes that we feel hot in, and honest relationships where we can be vulnerable, to a world where every child is safe, well-fed, and free.

—Mama Gena[1]

I can't do that. I can't change my diet. I can't leave him. I can't get off my meds. I can't wake up early. I can't move my body that way. I can't . . . I can't . . .

I can't is the mantra of a woman invested in the illusion of powerlessness. These words afford the familiar pleasure of opting out, giving up, and feeling constrained by a *No* that is imposed beyond your control. If you can't, then you'll never know the vulnerability of trying, of failing, or, even scarier, of boldly and audaciously changing your story.

There are the conscious *can'ts* and the subconscious *can'ts*. Subconscious *can'ts* are often found right beneath the disappointment, bitterness, and even hopelessness that attends the experience of *not having what you say you want.* These *can'ts* protect you from the learned risks of having more. When exposed, play-it-safe-and-small subconscious beliefs tend to sound more like:

I can't make more money. I can't take that risk. I can't be more powerful. I can't be more sensual. I can't be sexy. I can't be too beautiful, or confident, or unbothered. I can't have too much, have it too easy, or too exceptionally. No, no, I can't come out to play.

If your conscious *can'ts* keep you contracted into a familiar range of living, then your subconscious *can'ts* keep you safe from abandonment and betrayal, and the imagined punishment and consequences of expansion and growth. The prison guard keeping you locked in the too-small cell of possibility has noble intentions; however, your protectors can't actually keep you from your fears. They can only offer up a different menu of emotions such as numbness, irritation, and indignation. Your audacious adventure, the magic carpet ride of your womanly story, begins when you take one step and then another in the direction of your *I certainly can't have that!* unlived life.

Full and Wanting More

174

In so many ways, the marketing and advertising industries have commodified our own self-rejection and entrained feminine desire as a means of securing acceptance, approval, and relief from what is wrong inside. No wonder women are the target audience for all self-help and enhancement campaigns, and that we are exhausted from decades of performing and curating—rather than following our hearts.

Desire has a much more powerful and vital role to play in our lives than purchasing products or services. The deep desires, our life-defining voraciousness, can only be accessed when we practice being honest about *all* the desires that enter into our field of awareness. Desire is the organizing principle of creative impulse, arising from eros and generating connection between points, entities, humans, ideas, and structures that would otherwise remain disparate. Desire animates and vivifies. For a woman, desire is never-ending. You are never actually satiated, so it's best you develop a healthy intimate relationship with heart hunger. *She ain't goin' nowhere.*

David Deida describes the third-stage feminine as "full and wanting more." To want from fullness requires that you embrace what already exists, right here and now, and feel nourished, sustained, and fulfilled by what is, while also allowing for yearning to continue to bubble up from the depths.

Instead, most of us relate to desire in two stifled, constricted ways:

I don't *have* what I want.

I don't *know* what I want.

Finding Fullness:

I don't have what I want.

Yes, you do.

I would go so far as to say that you want exactly what you have, when you have it, and how you have it. An unseen part of you is being fulfilled by what you have and finds safety, familiarity, and maybe even pleasure in the apparent struggle with what is. These are called shadow desires and are essential to explore in the road beyond victim consciousness. Your shadow desires serve very legitimate parts of you (hint: your mother-wounded part who's used to attenuating and playing small) that don't actually want to be bigger, because that would put important people at risk of feeling uncomfortable, jealous, or bad about themselves. Exploring the upside of not having what you want is a humbling task, but it's also an empowering lifestyle and worldview. Never again will you experience random accidents, bad luck, or short ends of the stick. Your desire is restored at the helm of your ship.

I don't recommend getting lost in this exploration, however. This reframe is not intended to make you feel extra fucked-up for wishing misery on yourself. To my mind, knowing that a part of you is being fulfilled even as another part is feeling violated helps to expose the language of your patterns. It helps to illuminate why your struggles meet needs, and ultimately allows you to more consciously *choose* what is, in fact, occurring, with approval.

This is the fullness.

This is bringing a *Yes* to what was formerly a *No,* and I'm not sure there's a better way to do that than to unearth why your conscious complaints may be your unconscious wish list.

In fact, in the recesses of your desire vault, victim consciousness is pulsing strong. That victim consciousness has an unmitigated desire to be right about how wronged you are and finds the experience as enlivening as a Red Bull after a few nights of insomnia. It's a hit of life force in a desert of disconnection. I know this well from my days as a career activist, a truth warrior who said she wanted a better world for women and children, but who actually wanted every horrible mandate, false flag, and psyop predicted to come true. . . so that she could be right about how messed up everything is. On some, nearly impossible-to-acknowledge level, a part of me even wanted others to suffer at the hands of Pharma, so that I could have more proof of how wronged we are. And I needed the war to continue so that I could feel important and worthy.

One day, on stage, I told the story of a man who murdered his own son after having been started on Paxil for routine work stress. I could feel the rush of energy rise up my body as I transmitted this shocking, albeit true, Big Pharma exposé. I was claiming a bit of life-force, a hint of *Yes,* subconsciously, while pretending to myself and others that I was an unmitigated *No* to what I was sharing.

Gulp.

Exploring the full spectrum of wantingness requires that you visit with any and all hidden intentions to learn what you might be enjoying about the things you consciously reject. Very kinky, indeed.

Once you realize that you want what you hate, what you have, and what is, you can feel the fullness and begin to invite authentic yearning into the arena. How can you make what you're reluctantly doing (because you don't *have* to do *anything*) more pleasurable?

If you can't get out of it, get into it.

Commuting? Find an amazing podcast like Reclamation Radio to listen to. Making dinner for one? Put on music and take out the fine china. Struggling with your husband? Focus on his amazing attributes and express appreciation just to throw a curve ball.

Often, we draw a blank when invited to shift from what we hate to what we actually want. We've been so focused on our complaints that we have not taken one moment to explore what *is* wanted.

Wanting more:

I don't know what I want.

Many of us have cut ourselves off entirely from wanting, moving through life disconnected from the banquet of desire, accepting crumbs from complaint. We are unwilling to admit what we want (due to shame, guilt, limited permission field, spiritual bypassing) or because we've preemptively decided that what we want is simply unrealistic. Because we get tripped up by how complicated or impossible it would be to have the thing we want, we dismiss our known desires as fantasy, and we go on tolerating what we don't want. Whether you're complaining about your health, your relationship, your finances, or your employees, I promise there is a seedling of vulnerable desire that wants to grow.

I believe that you do know what you want, because you know what you don't want.

Your complaints are portals to desire.

So, give your victim the mic and let her expound upon the injustices in your lifescape: What are your biggest complaints in business, in love, in mothering, in finances, with the world? Beneath every complaint is a desire. When you have identified what is unwanted— *the neighbor is too loud*—you now know that you want quiet. When you feel strung out and spread too thin, you want spaciousness and ease, or maybe support and simplicity.

Maybe you complain that your friend is so disrespectful and always late. Beneath your complaint is the desire to feel honored, to matter, and to feel cared for. Meanwhile, your friend is late for her own reasons that likely have nothing to do with you, yet it can feel delicious to judge her tardiness as personal, and terrifying to express with vulnerability that you want to feel that she loves you enough to show up on time. Desire is a tender thing for you to protect and steward.

As we get to know desire within us, we might only choose to see her light side. Her sweet longing for a loving partner, the sufficient bank account, and maybe that pink silk dress in the window. Desire is prismatic and complicated, just like you, and as you go deeper with her, you'll learn about desires beneath the surface of those modest wants. You'll learn about taboo and naughty desires, even shameful ones, and beyond those are the desires for things to be hard, fucked up, and exactly how they *actually are*.

I've observed that desire comes in three flavors: apologetic, acceptable, and audacious. (I'll never miss an opportunity for alliteration.)

Apologetic desires:

These live in the realm of shame and the illusion that if you don't acknowledge a desire, it doesn't exist. However, unacknowledged desires seep out as condemning vitriol, judgment, and envy. So, when you are self-reflective, honest, and real about what you want and why, everyone wins.

For example, maybe you want to feel exquisitely taken care of or served. Maybe you want to be a housewife and stay at home with your kids (which feels shameful because you were raised by a good feminist mommy). Maybe you want to frolic around in a forest all damn day. Maybe you want to run a bakery that only employs shirtless male models, and the vision came to you in a flash on a random Wednesday.

But these desires feel irrational, unreasonable, or embarrassing. An inner protector delivers tirades like:

What's wrong with you? What kind of woman wants to be alone when she chooses to have children?!

Or: *How dare you wish away your opportunity to work and make a living?! A kept woman? What is this, the 1950s?!*

You judge women who are doing these things, trolling their social media profiles and crusading for your enlightened perspectives on how women should act. You keep *should*ing yourself into the reality you deem appropriate, and you hustle for promotions when you'd rather arrange mandalas from the flowers you collected in the garden.

What's fascinating to me is that an honest exploration of a taboo life desire often leads to a refinement of the desire and clarity around its root driver. You may have trouble admitting that you've thought longingly about a divorce, but if you actually invite that desire to sit with you over tea, you might learn that what's even deeper in the hidden realms is the desire for connection, attention, and safety from the very man you secretly fantasize about leaving. We simply can't know if we won't look.

Acceptable desires:

These desires are polite, demure, and socially tame.

Does this sound familiar? A colleague of mine recently shared: "You know, Kelly, I'm stuck in this financial thing. I don't need to make tons of money or anything, I just want to have enough money to travel." I told her straight up, "That sounds terrible. Enough money 'just to travel'? That bar feels un-limbo-ably low."

The easiest way to smoke out a virtue-signaling acceptable desire is to deliver the simple inquiry: Why?

I want my business to be successful, but I want my offerings to be accessible.

Why?

The real answer is because that's what a good girl is allowed to want. To want or ask for more than your allotment of crumbs would be so unspiritual of you!

Once you know why you want that acceptable thing, is that really all you want, or might there be more that you want just for you?

The thing that the acceptable desire doesn't realize is this: what you truly want is actually best for everyone else around you as well. When you get raw and real with yourself about what you want, it organizes every aspect of your lifescape into coherence because you are now aligned with you, freeing everyone around you to do the same.

Enter: Audacious wants!

Former dominatrix and Taoist nun, Kasia Urbaniak, penned one of the most game-changing books I've ever read (and that's saying something) on the subject of audacious wants, encouraging women to go big and bold with their wildest desires. *Unbound* teaches women how to unlock the power of imagination to live into the world we've not yet permitted ourselves to inhabit. When we want big, we might shock ourselves with what's uncorked.

An audacious want may be to open an elevated mocktail bar, or an all-female owned and operated exotic dance club, or a full-service psychiatric medication taper holistic retreat center . . . okay, those are *my* audacious wants. I could come up with a long list of reasons why those are fabulous, meaningful, and important ideas, but the truth is that I just want to do those things because I want to. And they also feel crazy to want because who do I think I am wanting those things? In order to keep the channel of wanting open and unmitigated, your wants need to feel welcome, not interrogated for reasons they deserve to exist.

David Deida encourages women to speak from this achy place of heart yearning and helplessness as a practice. He says that women learn self-sufficiency in what he calls the second stage (our *No* phase) and then can *choose* to experience vulnerability, softness, and even helplessness in the third stage. Helplessness is a flavor of the feminine that attracts caretaking, protectorship, and guardianship from the masculine (your own and others'); it's what makes a man feel needed, worthy, and important in the dyad. He uses the example of how a woman in an old movie might approach a puddle. The man near her won't put his coat down over the puddle if she puts down her own, yet he is invited to offer her this care if she expresses third-stage helplessness through her body as the longing for his devotion. She doesn't need it; she deeply wants it. When you arrive at this stage in your actualization, your masculine is online and you *can* take care of yourself as a woman, but it can hurt to have to. So, speaking from this achy place, from the helpless place, from the longing that never left but was shored up through independence, can represent a reconnection to God through the opening of your body vessel.

Finding moments in the day to practice speaking from that ache of helplessness, just infusing whatever it is that you might otherwise say with an open, soft, expectant energy, can integrate desire into an otherwise dry landscape of doing and fixing.

The Art of Asking for What You Want

In addition to helping us claim wild desires, Kasia Urbaniak outlines tools to get our energy coherent and attention directed through what she calls the dominant and submissive ask. Templated by her BDSM experience, Urbaniak knows that the needs of two people can be complementary when roles are delineated and intentions clarified, and that skilled communication is essential to actualize these potentialities. All that is required is that you know what you want and who can help you get it. Urbaniak teaches women how to intentionally assume either the dominant or submissive energy before making a coherently articulated ask, and this alignment short-circuits the good girl conditioning that keeps us in the middle ground we occupy when we are afraid to be too bitchy or too needy.

For example, imagine you say to your partner, "It would be great if you could plan an evening for once." Not unlike harshly demanding a hug, this mixed energy is at the root of so much relational unfulfillment, conflict, and tension.

So how do you ask for what you want?

The dominant ask is about holding your attention *out*: it's direct, other-focused, crisp, and clear. It tells a person what to do, perhaps even when and how to do it. And if that dominant energy, for whatever reason, does not receive what it's asking for, there's no recoil or contraction. Attuned and focused, the good Domme locates the source of resistance and puts words to it, navigating with alacrity.

Let's imagine that you're looking to launch a sticker business, and you need roughly $1,000 to get it off the ground. You know your uncle is good for the money, and you decide to ask from your dominant energy. You might say something like, "My new business needs funding to the tune of 1,000 bucks. You're just the man to make it happen."

The submissive ask, on the other hand, is focused *inward* and is an invitation into the desire made manifest through the heroic role of the person being asked. The submissive ask requires that you, as the asker, vivify the fantasy of what you want and that you invite your subject into the dream state of this desire. Asking from this energy, you are giving him the opportunity to make your dreams come true. So, in the same situation as above, a Sub ask would sound something like, "I've had this dream to start an online awakened sticker company since I was little, and I feel like it's finally time to make this dream a reality. I need $1,000 to get this business onto its feet. You have always been a hero in my life, and I would feel like a princess being carried off to the castle if you could help me. Will you?"

Or, back to our dinner request; instead of saying, "Let's go to dinner!" or "You wanna go out to dinner?" you could journey there, in your felt imagination—the music, the lighting, the taste of the first bite, the laughter bubbling up from inside you, his gaze from across the table, your silk dress—and you could invite him to make this happen—all of it—in the way that only he can. "I love the way I feel when you take me out for dinner," or "I've had such an incredible time going to restaurants with you, I would so love it if . . . " Speaking from your felt experience is what draws people *in*; it's an alluring and irresistible way to co-create with the perfect person.

Know what you want. Ask for it with intentionality. Watch desires become reality.

PRACTICE THE SUBMISSIVE ASK

The next time you want something and are ready to ask for it, play with the submissive ask.

Dinner with a girlfriend	Remember that time we went for drinks and tapas and ended up having the most amazing evening? I'd love to recreate that magic with you next Thursday. Are you down?
Borrowing your neighbor's car	I need your help because my car broke down and I have a million things to do. I would have such peace of mind if I knew I could borrow your car for a few hours. It would feel like I have family that I can count on. Will you?
Asking your friends to help you pack	I'm totally stumped on what to pack and you guys have the best fashion advice! I'd feel like a runway model being dressed to walk if you'd come over to help me pick some things out.
Requesting financial support to sign up for a new program	There's a fantastic opportunity coming up that could make a major impact in my future, and I need your support to make this dream a reality. Will you donate to my audacious future fund?

Havingness

You may think that you want to live in bliss forever more, but you probably couldn't even handle a blissful Monday (let alone a blissful life), and neither can I. If you've ever touched unadulterated ecstasy, be it through lovemaking or plant medicine or deep meditation, then you'll know that it's obliterating to fully hold and receive, even for ten seconds. If expanding to hold transcendent states requires a sound and resourced nervous system, then titration into deep okayness, pleasure, and fulfillment is a sort of early courtship phase of this inner relationship.

Before I made a regular practice of the Deepest Fear Inventory (which I'll detail below), I thought that all of me wanted to work less, be more supported in my business, and make more money. But then, despite my best intentions, I would continue to work more and hit a revenue ceiling. I had even sprinkled in some manifestation practices, like feeling into how delicious that softpreneur life would be, a few affirmations, and some envisioning sessions with my team. What I didn't know then was that there was a part of me that felt safe and connected when I could complain about my business, hard work, and all the things that were going wrong.

In my sessions with my erotic coach, Whitney, I started prioritizing my pleasure, slowing down, resting, and playing more. During the first year after my second marriage ended, I told myself that my business was failing because I was single for the first time in my life, and it was too hard to do it all. I told myself this for nine whole months. I complained and whined about my victim story about the struggles with my launches, expenses, and disappointing vendors to anyone who would listen. Until a P&L was requested by a consultant and I saw in black and white that by September of that year, I had already brought in over a million dollars, on my own. It wasn't safe (for all of me) to acknowledge this expansion and to live in that largess, so I told myself a smalling story that felt safer and kept me swirling in the stimulation of frustration.

After this jolt, I began to practice celebrating to expand my havingness capacity.

I decided to tell the truth about these wins to a few girlfriends, each of whom was struggling financially, and I survived it. In fact, they celebrated along with me. No punishment, no consequences, no alienation. The next step was for me to begin to do what I'm doing right now, which is to own the success and fulfillment of my business publicly, as an activist whose career has been founded on wrestling rather than enjoying life.

And I continued to learn more about my divided will around having an easeful, abundant life in the process. In fact, I got a bit of unsolicited feedback recently when I was promoting a workshop on the psychospirituality of business called Audacious Entrepreneurship. This gal commented online:

> *Basically she's admitting that she unethically makes an obscene amount of money for almost no work at all. And sits there priding herself on it. Yet there are people who work 60+ hours a week and can't even afford groceries.*

185

It bothered me, and I could have cooked up quite a scathing reply about her unacknowledged desire for exactly what I have masquerading as virtuous caretaking of the anonymous victim. Instead, I entered through the upset and found the part of me that also believes I shouldn't have wealth unless I am trading my life, that I can't expand without punishment, and that I need to justify my havingness through rationale, guilt, and apology.

Interestingly, that very day, a woman had complimented my hair, and specifically my curls, after a Pilates class. Instead of receiving with a *Thank you!* I said, *Thanks! It's a lot of work.*

Huh?!

It was Attenuator-in-chief that was tasked with making sure this woman felt comfortable with my beauty: beauty that's apparently so burdensome, she shouldn't want it, anyway. Safe, connected, relatable, small. Well done! Because beautiful, easy hair is not what I actually want. Beautiful, difficult hair: okay, I can work with that.

When havingness is coupled with unsafety, we have an opportunity to show ourselves that here, in this adult woman's life, safety can be generated from within, one small experience of having more at a time.

Think of what follows as an all-out desire manifestation map to discover, own, and explore your uncharted, audacious desires; because when it comes to desire, more is decidedly more. A woman's desire makes the world, after all. Time to offer your Godspark to the fire of creation.

I. FEEL IT
FIND THE PLEASURE IN THE UPSET

Express the Shape Your Body Wants to Make
Inspired by my erotic coach, Whitney
Pleasure hunting is how I like to honor the feelings in my body, and it turns out that there is pleasure in the shapes the body wants to take when feeling difficult feels.

Through subtle urges and impulses, the body is trying to tell you "This would feel better if I could just move in this way!"

If this energy/emotion could take over your body, what would it have you do? Throw a tantrum and stomp around with exasperation? Shake the "I'm scared" out of your bones? Surrender to the shame and curl into a ball?

Let your feelings lead and take you over from face to feet. This doesn't have to be a Broadway performance. The important thing is to keep moving, but slooooow it down. Play with gestures and postures to embody what you're feeling, and move for the enjoyment of it.

When you've created a container to feel what is there to feel, ask your body what shape she wants to take. Move into that gesture or position slowly, watching for any aspect of the movement that, itself feels pleasurable.

When you listen to your body, pleasure is a natural consequence, even if you are listening to what she wants to do with a painful feeling.

FEEL THE LONGING:

What do you *know* that you want? Like *sooo* bad. But you don't have it yet . . . and maybe you never will, or maybe it will come tomorrow, but it feels like you can't live one more second without it? It could be a dream partner, a miraculous windfall of money, an inconceivable cure, a life-changing opportunity, anything that you can almost *taste* . . .

Isolate that feeling of yearning and experience it only as a pure longing, uncoupled from the cover emotions of bitterness, fear, and vigilant problem-solving. When I have sat with longing, it feels like a freight train tunneling through my core, and I often have to pendulate to a distal region that is sensation-free just to experience relief for a few seconds.

Sit comfortably and allow your body to take the shape of longing for thirty to ninety seconds. No story. Just feeling.

FEEL THE FULLNESS:

Take seventeen seconds to feel the *yes*!

Find a feeling about anything delightful, big or small, in your life. Let the fullness saturate your entire body with luminous energy, filling you from head to toe, and as you give it your full and appreciative attention, let the sensation expand out beyond your skin like radiant joy.

Make a practice of pausing in this way throughout the day and seize every opportunity to receive when you note something delightful, even if mundane. That radiant glow will follow you wherever you go as you condition yourself to live in delicious appreciation and train your eyes to see the *yes*.

II. FACE IT
EXISTENTIAL KINK

An Adaptation of Carolyn Lovewell's Deepest Fear Inventory

Sometimes, the only thing standing in your way is you pretending to hate the thing you have and to feel forsaken in your unrequited longing for the thing you don't have. When we make our fears conscious, we can validate, feel, and honor them, and desire can be liberated into more audacious expressions.

One of my favorite tools for exploring unconscious fears and associated desires starts with a simple journal prompt:

"I absolutely refuse to have *[fill in the blank with what you claim to want]* because I have a deep fear that I . . ."

The answer to why you don't have what you want lies in the answer to that statement.

Let's use wealth as an example.

Many people wish to have all the money because it would lead to financial independence. With that kind of dough, alarm clocks become a thing of the past, vacations happen all year round, and life feels beautiful.

BUT what if there were downsides to having that kind of wealth? I mean, mo' money, mo' problems, right? Like people always judging you for not being generous enough, no matter how much you give, or criminals looking to take advantage of your kind nature? You might even be afraid that you'll mismanage your wealth and lose it all, only to feel worse than you did before you ever lived the rich life.

If a part of you is terrified of having money, that part of you is getting exactly what she wants when you don't have it.

So here's how you do it:

- Write *I absolutely refuse to have [this thing I say I want] because I have a deep fear that I will* . . . at the top of a page.

- List out as many things as come to mind in five minutes of writing.
- Read this out loud (extra points for reading to a friend).
- Then burn it.

Do this same exercise on the same topic, every day for a week, until it gets boring and you've seen what there is to see about the many reasons you don't entirely want the thing you say you want, and why your struggle is actually just what the doctor ordered.[2]

SHE'S GOT IT, I WANT IT

Every single one of us has someone in our lives who rubs us the wrong way, and this exercise is about girl-on-girl hate crimes. Think about a woman in your lifescape that drives you nuts.

- **What is it about her that you can't stand, disgusts you, or raises your alarms?** Does she speak her opinions too freely, wear clothes you find scandalous, or even just seem too happy given the state of things?
- **What are you making it mean about her as a woman?** What is true about her because she does those terrible things?
- **What dire and fully deserved consequences should she face because of her choices?** Should she be ostracized from your group of friends, forced into etiquette training, or become the focus of gossipy rhetoric?
- **Who do you get to be because she is this way?** Who are you relative to her? If someone were looking at the two of you and your respective behaviors, what would they say about her and what would they say about you?
- **What would it be like if you could be just a little like her—without consequences?** Would you sit on the couch a little longer? Would you speak like you had

something important to say? Would you wear the tighter dress?

- **What would you want to take on if you could magically have some aspects of what she's up to?** Would you be more popular? Have more money? Be sexier? Have more answers? Make a better pie?
- **Do you imagine there are some aspects of who and how *you are* that she might admire, appreciate, or want to emulate?** Maybe she sees you as free-spirited and creative. Or maybe she admires your steadiness under pressure while she seems to loudly bumble through scenarios like the quirky friend in a sitcom. What would you appreciate about yourself through her eyes?

The point is that on the other side of your judgments is often a sneaky shadow side of longing. So, take a look at those ladies who rub you the wrong way and see if they aren't trying to show you that maybe you *want* to be a little more like them—if only you dared!

RESOLVE IF/THEN LIVING
STEP INTO AUDACIOUS DESIRE

My coach Whitney taught me this reflective exercise to resolve the trap of thinking that I can only have what I want once a certain goal is met, when, in actuality, I can use the imagined fulfillment of my desires to point me toward the ways in which I already have what I want.

Take a minute to ponder what your life will look like once all your desires are fulfilled. Let's say your goal is to have a strong, masculine man who doesn't collapse when you feel all your big, audacious feelings. Were that goal achieved, consider the following:

Who do you get to be with that man?

- Do you get to feel more feminine, allowed to explore and experience the full spectrum of female emotions without fear of censorship or rejection?
- Do you get to feel fully wanted in all your facets?

What do you get to _do_?
- Do you get to follow his lead, surrendering to his guidance because you trust him to hold you safely in his masculine container?
- Are you free to express your emotions in bigger, healthier ways?
- Do you feel more authentic in your expressions?

What do you get to _have_?
- Do you get to feel safe and secure?
- When you feel safe, do you finally feel like you can surrender?
- Do you feel _free_?

Now, explore how you could start embodying these things and living that life _before_ you actually achieve your goal. How can you live the dream _now_, so you aren't waiting around for one thing to happen before you can achieve the other?

How can you feel more feminine and pleasure-led _now_?
- Dance how you might if you had an audience.
- Adorn yourself how you imagine he'd prefer (which would, of course, be what lights _you_ up and makes _you_ shine with inner fire).
- Incorporate the touch of a four-handed massage.
- Sit in nature and enjoy a moment of serenity with a cup of tea.
- Purge your closet and home of things that make you feel drab and sparkless.

How can you give up the lead so you can feel more authentic and fully expressed _now_?
- Where can you delegate tasks and share workload?
- Where can you give up leadership around the house?
- Are there "I can do it myself" habits that are more draining than they need to be?
- Can you hire out some of the adulting, so you have more time to be _you_?

What could you do *now* to feel more authentic and fully expressed?

- Where are you diluting your truth? Where are you dimming your own expression? Where does it feel safe to let go and be completely real for once?
- Ask friends to gather for a ritual to honor your Reclaimed Woman era.
- Organize a fun event, like a private erotic dance lesson in your own home with a few close girlfriends.
- Curate a meeting of minds with people who get fired up about the same things you do.

What can you do to feel safer *now*?

- Could you increase security at your home with locks and maybe even a camera or two?
- Can you identify a check-in buddy who says goodnight each night?
- Can you work with a somatic experiencing practitioner to help you find safety in your body?

192

The key is to practice receiving what you want via feeling it.

So, for example, if you adorn yourself like a woman who's in love, notice where you feel the pleasure of that in your body. Practice feeling it for just three breaths at a time, like a body-based meditation. If thoughts distract you from feeling the pleasure, you can shake it out (rather than think it out) or tense your whole body and release, before returning to feeling the pleasure again.

Ground into the idea that it's not just about DOING these things, it's about BEING in the experiences you want by anchoring into the pleasure for a few breaths, taking a break (shaking, tense and release, etc.), then coming back to the pleasure.

As you practice embodying the real results of your goals, you'll be better prepared for when you actually achieve it, so you don't get trapped in the underwhelm of getting everything you ever wanted. You're already living as the main character of your audacious life, right now.[3]

THE VICTIM AND THE ANTHROPOLOGIST

When I announced the ending of my second marriage, I wrote "it had to be this way," and trust me when I say that ending that relationship felt like waking up out of anesthesia intraoperative.

But I've said before and I'll say again: suffering ends where meaning begins.

So, let's practice sovereign meaning-making:

Why did your most shitty, horrible, no-fair-why-me experience NEED to happen?

- First tell the story from your victim, complete with all the vitriol, blaming, disgust, and rage.
- Then tell the story from your inner anthropologist. You know, the one who has been studying your life and who has the big-picture version of events.

How can you make sense of why you wanted it to be this way? What did you get to feel that was old, stuck, and wanting release? What contrast was provided as you moved from turmoil to treasure?

III. FREE IT
EXPAND INTO HAVINGNESS

Since our lives are incredibly fast-paced, we do many things on autopilot, even things we enjoy. When sex becomes routine, and pleasure gets lost in schedules and commitments, it can be hard to recognize opportunities to just take a minute and sloooow the fuck down so you can spend a bit of time just allowing yourself to feel *really good*. It's possible to take time for simple tasks of self-care and turn them into moments of divinely sensual self-devotion. I firmly believe that women in healed alliance with their own desires have the capacity to shape the direction of the collective in a way that can bring into manifestation that which we couldn't otherwise imagine, but sometimes baby steps are essential to begin to heal the disconnection from our own bodies and impulses.

Here are a few ways you can downshift into a pleasure pace, even if it's just for a minute:

1. **Brush your hair like a lover would.** Feel the brush as it scratches and stimulates your scalp. Enjoy the repetitive strokes and luxuriate in the feel of the silky strands detangling under your fingers.
2. **Put on lotion.** Apply lotion like it's a benediction, a practice of self-devotion that goes much deeper than the skin. Massage your sore muscles, smooth your hands over your dry elbows and weary feet. Feel the moisture sink into your skin as your self-love sinks into your soul.
3. **Stand in a ray of sunlight.** Like a cat in the window, just allow yourself to bask, and revel in the warmth on your face, the peace in your mind, and the fact that you're allowed to set aside even ten seconds to enjoy the simple and sensual pleasure of sunshine.
4. **Enjoy every bite.** When eating can feel like a practice of shoving food into your mouth hole as you run about your busy life, it can be incredibly grounding to sit down, turn off your distractions like cell phones, TVs, and even other people, and mindfully enjoy a meal. No clock, no pressure, no expectations: just you and some delicious food.
5. **Just dance.** Turn on the music and let it tell your body how to move, without audience or self-censorship. Sway, twirl, sing, shake, and writhe. Don't dance like nobody's watching; dance like

you're watching, and you're the most important audience in the world.

6. **Five minutes of what she wants.** Set a timer for five minutes (or start with three), lie in your bed, and feel what your body wants. Do that. Then feel again. Then do that. Maybe she wants socks on. More air conditioning. Your hands to rub your neck. Maybe a gentle stroking on your inner thigh or a squeeze of your forearm. Listen and then offer.

7. **Breast massage.** A cardinal devotional practice, breast massage can be a beautiful self-offering. I use my friend Isa of Pelvic Pain Relief's oil, called B Healthy, in the shower. With intuitive sweeps, I enjoy the softness of this sacred center on my body, not for my health per se, but because it feels good.

Find the already present pleasures in your body and apply yourself to them with all the worship you'd normally save for the divine.

FREE MONEY SHOPPING LIST

Shared by Kasia Urbaniak, this game helps define genuine wants and clarify havingness ceilings, and it reminds us that it's okay to feature ourselves in our fantasies. Here's how you play:

1. List everything you'd buy, today, if you had infinite cash flow. This isn't like that grocery game show where everyone heads to the meat section first. Get creative! Go to real estate websites, order a yacht, buy VIP tickets, plan the European five-star tour with friends, and finally hit Checkout on every Wish List you've ever created. Everything has to be for you to have—not for charity, gifts, or resale.

2. Search for the prices and add up the total value of all your material wants.

Creating Versus Fixing

Since fixing implies that there is something "bad" or inherently "wrong" with you, someone else, or with reality, the impulse to fix keeps you trapped inside a loop of "never enough" and insists that your energy be funneled toward controlling external circumstances. When you're stuck in fixing, your gaze is focused in the opposite direction of what you wish to create, moving you closer to the issue at hand instead of further away from it. When you're fixing, your work is in healing your flaws.

But the real magic lies in *creating*, because you marry your desire to the here and now. Engaging in creating entails embodying the version of you that you wish to live into, rather than incessantly chasing a dangling carrot you can never seem to catch. When you prioritize creating over fixing, you shed defensiveness and righteousness, and you no longer take the bait of provocation because you have your gaze trained on what feels good rather than glaring at what's hated.

I profoundly shifted my focus from fixing to creating in 2015, after the death of my mentor, Nick Gonzalez, left me questioning everything. From the depths of my grief, I felt for the North Star of my own heart and recognized that the only part of my mission, my vocation, and my day-to-day that I actually enjoyed were the dogma-defying stories of health reclamation, not ardently fighting vaccine mandates.

It was the triumph, the alchemy, the *Yes* spun from a *No* in the women I worked with that opened my vessel and brought tears to my eyes. So, I aligned with that truth, and focused my energy on *what is possible* rather than *what is wrong*. I assembled a team of volunteers and published history-making papers, including a clinical trial demonstrating that radical healing is possible through basic lifestyle change. So, in 2020, when new mandates met my sovereign unmasked self, I assembled a team to catalyze a grassroots event called the Thank You Body Rally (thankyoubodyrally.com) that would bring a hundred locations together across the world in celebration of the body's capacity to heal, complete with music, art, dance, and merriment.

Fight the problem dangling in front of you or find the joy already here. Are you fixing or are you creating? As you heal your relationship with desire, creating will become the irresistible choice.

CHAPTER 13

Erotic Artistry

Who's Touching Who & Why

Eros is what will restore our fragmented world. This embodied life force energy is the expression of the divine impulse, born of pleasure and the desire to create what can't be created and nourished through control and force-based power. It flows between us and weaves us into the fabric of our nature. At its core, eros needs consent and willingness to thrive, to preserve the flow of life force energy, and can't exist within the polarity energies of domination, deception, and parasitism. It can be stifled so easily by outside influence, and in order to reclaim the eros energy within you, you need to be incredibly clear on what you allow into your life and be very aware of how others try to impose their will on your divine spark.

As an attentive and capable custodian of your vital force energy, you're ready to start setting safe containers for pleasure and play. And if you're like me, you'll be astounded by how many decades you've lived in this body, disconnected and unaware of the pleasure that is available when the performing and appeasing stop and conscious presence and intention are prioritized.

When you get clear on what you want and how to ask for it, you'll notice how many experiences in life involve giving what you assume is wanted, taking without asking, and allowing without really wanting to, and how much pleasure is left on the table. In the dynamics of desire, consent smokes out any unacknowledged intentions; when you understand who is doing what to whom and for what reason, all sorts of pleasure and safety become possible.

Like a skilled dance instructor arriving to a class full of tripping, flailing, toe-stomping dancers, Betty Martin is here to demonstrate what is possible through two people moving with intention, clarity, and permission. A long-time sex educator, Betty shares a spectacular model that breaks down the many nuanced layers of giving and receiving. She calls this model "the wheel of consent," and once explored, you will never look at touch the same way again.

Consent goes so much further than the transaction itself; it's a practice of knowing yourself, loving yourself, and familiarizing yourself with your deeply held desires, so you can engage with the desires of another person and find the complementarity therein. There are countless ways we've societally numbed out to the point of not even recognizing the sensory organ that is the body, such as the old world "gatekeeper" models of sexual consent, where a man wants sex, the woman has the sex, and it's his job to go out there and get it from her. There is so much "going with the flow," performing, mind reading, and misattunement that can be resolved through clarified intention and expression of desire.

For example, imagine there's a hand moving across your body, but explicit consent hasn't been communicated. The hand may believe he is giving touch and pleasure while the body may believe she is giving pleasure to the hand by offering herself, or that her pleasure is pleasurable to the hand-bearer. Who is actually receiving pleasure here, and how?

Martin so brilliantly breaks down this model of consent into four quadrants, where one person is "doing," one is being "done to," and the axis on the wheel is divided into giving and receiving.

Diagram[1]

Doing

Consent

Yes, I will . . .

SERVE   TAKE

action   action

gift

gift

ALLOW   ACCEPT

Giving
(it's for them)

Receiving
(it's for me)

Will you . . . ?

Done to

Doing

In the old paradigm, the person doing is the person giving, simple as that. However, in the wheel of consent, the person doing could be either giving or receiving, depending on the consensual agreement (more on that below).

Done to

Similar to the one doing, when you're being "done to," you're either *receiving* touch in the way you'd like, or you're giving the gift of your bodily access, *letting* yourself be done to.

You can see here how *both* the acts of "doing" and being "done to" can operate simultaneously. The one doing can be giving a gift to the receiver, or receiving access to them in some way, which is a gift to themselves. Same goes for the one receiving, where they can be receiving that touch just the way they would like or be giving access to their body at that moment in time. This is where the other quadrants come in, bringing even more real-world nuance.

Serving & Taking

Existing within the "doing" quadrant, one could be doing for the benefit of the other (serving) or doing for your own benefit (taking). The Server says "Yes, I will," in response to a request he/she is willing to offer for the benefit of the other, as in giving a massage, while the Taker says, "May I?" to express a desire that he/she has to touch another's body. Most of us only know taking touch in the form of petting a cat or dog, but we covertly take touch while pretending to give touch all the time with our partners. To take from your lover is to ravish, and when that desire isn't acknowledged, allowed, and honored, a shamewall is erected (pun intended) and undercover operations commence.

Allow & Accept

Falling under the "done to" category, these two actions are receptive in nature, but operate differently. When you're allowing, you're *giving*, as you're granting access to a part of you for the benefit of another (e.g., allowing someone to caress the small of your back). The phrase Betty pairs with allowing is "Yes, you may," as you're giving the person asking *access* to you (the gift they get to receive). Accepting on the other hand, is paired with the question "Will you?" as it's directly related to the thing you *want* to have happen, as in "Will you rub my feet?"

201

What's so epically revolutionary about Betty Martin's wheel of consent practice is that it creates a platform, not just for agency, boundaries, and assertive communication, but also for your right to pleasure.[2]

Just think about how many relationships exist that are predicated on *many* years of transactional interactions, assumed mutual satisfaction, and a narrow sexual repertoire. Sexual sovereignty becomes possible when you can wholeheartedly meet yourself in the field of desire, where you can hear your body's wisdom, what it's deeply longing for, and then finally ask for what you want. This approach confers true safety to an otherwise potentially perilous realm of sensuality and sexuality. Finally, you can move energy through specific channels of desire with your partner while identifying where his wants intersect with your wants, your willing to's, and your unwilling to boundaries. There are new dimensions of play and pleasure that become available when you learn first who is doing what for whom, how to ask for it, and where your actual limits lie.

As Martin beautifully elucidates: "It's huge work to personally identify how you would want to touch someone's body, or to have your body be touched. That open eye consent experience, that agreement where you know it's safe because they are willing and you can trust their willingness, is such a powerful rewiring, and it involves receiving on both ends of that wheel."[3]

RECLAMATION REMEDY: TURN ON YOUR SKIN

The 3-Minute Game, adapted from Betty Martin (invented by Harry Faddis)

This exercise centers on only two questions explored with a known or unknown partner, clothed or not. The first question:

"How do you want *me to touch you* for three minutes?" Here are a few possibilities:

- I'd like to put my head in your lap and have you massage my scalp, but gently, without pulling my hair.
- I'd like you to massage my scalp, but scratch with your fingernails and every now and then take large handfuls of my hair and pull them with traction.
- I'd like you to press your body weight onto me by laying on top of me, squishing me.
- I'd like you to gently tap my face and chest with your fingertips while I close my eyes and breathe deeply.
- I'd like you to massage my feet, rotating my ankles and pulling on my big toes.

- I'd like you to squeeze my legs, from my calves up to my thighs.

You might be totally down for what they want, or you might find that some aspect of their request doesn't align with your wants or willing to's. Negotiate what feels comfortable for both of you, then set a timer and spend the next three minutes giving them the requested touch.

Next, you're going to ask them, "How would *you like to touch me?*"

Many people have never been asked what they'd like to do to another person, and it can feel very vulnerable to ask for permission to do what you truly want. In this exercise, you're allowing them to freely and fully express how they want to touch you, knowing it's safe and that you're allowed to create boundaries around their wants as they pertain to your own body.

They might say things like:

- I want to explore the soft skin of your neck and shoulders.
- I want to run my hands through your hair and grab it in a ponytail.
- I want to press my face into your neck, chest, and abdomen.
- I want you to straddle my waist while seated so I can hug your body and rest my head in your chest.

Look inside yourself and ask, *Is what they want something that I can give them **that's a full YES for me?***

Negotiate what feels good and right for both of you, then set the timer and spend three minutes exploring what they've asked you for. Notice as you flow through the fields of giving, taking, doing, and receiving.

Take turns asking these questions of each other and deepen your field of permission. When it comes time to explore this exercise with a romantic or sexual partner, you'll be much more comfortable asking for what you want, and they'll be much more comfortable sharing with you what they want.

It all begins with three minutes and two simple questions.[4]

Bossy Massage, Adapted from an Exercise by Betty Martin

Bossy Massage is another amazing tool that I have even practiced with my daughters over the years. In this exercise, the receiver slows down enough to notice what is wanted and to ask for it. It can feel vulnerable to have a ready servant, on standby to give you exactly what you want—within their own comfortable boundaries, of course. But there's value to both sides of the transaction, with the receiver getting what they asked for, and the giver learning more about service without assuming what's wanted. The container of the Bossy Massage is designed to prevent the receiver from slipping into allowing, tolerating, or enduring energy and to prevent the giver from mindreading and creative interpretation of requests.

So how do you get (and give!) a Bossy Massage?

1. The receiver gets comfortable on a massage table, choosing her own positioning, and is given the option of a blanket if she'd prefer to be covered. Clothing is also optional, and the giver and receiver can discuss their own boundaries and comfort levels around how much, if any, clothing is required.

   While Bossy Massage can be very sexy if both parties are consenting, it can also be incredibly innocent and pure. As the receiver settles in, the giver waits, allowing her time to check in with her body and see what kind of touch she wants.

2. Without feeling pressured to say something or to blurt out the first thing that comes to your mind,

take time to really consider what it is that you want from this experience, and wait for what you actually want to become clear. What kind of touch would you like to feel? Be precise and specific. Once you know what you want, keep directing until you get it. Be a bossy bitch, respectfully.

Examples of types of touch: squeeze, stroke, tap, poke, rub, heavy pressure, light pressure, pet, grab. Some people want to be laid upon, using the giver as a human blanket. Anything is fair game for the receiver to request, and for the giver to consent to offer.

3. Once a Bossy request has been made and both parties are comfortable that their boundaries are met, the giver touches the receiver exactly how they're told, often with slight adjustments as the giver asks, "Like this?" to clarify the request further. The giver checks in frequently, and after thirty seconds steps away from the receiver, awaiting a new request.

4. Continue like this, with the receiver being Bossy and purposeful in their requests, and the giver patiently holding space for and fulfilling those requests, both openly communicating around comfort levels. Once your predetermined amount of time, say twenty minutes, is up, you thank each other for sharing this Bossy time, and everyone goes about their day.

It can take several sessions to feel truly comfortable just giving a clear command, and some things are more difficult to ask for than others. Don't be surprised if lots of feelings come up, even tears. It's incredibly challenging being Bossy with your desires when you've never been given the opportunity to just say what you want. This exercise takes the paradigm of *touch is something that happens to me* and completely turns it upside down. You'll also want to be mindful of what Martin describes as "asking side-ways for what you want"—where you may find yourself asking in a way that suggests, "Well, you could do this," or "Would you please, maybe, do this?" Martin explains, "There's nothing wrong with that—we all have different habits, but we want to gradually move from where we are into being just a little bit more bossy."[5]

Waking Up the Hands
As our Handless Maiden has shown, our hands nurture, they sense, they create, and they spring forth from the heart; here's another game-changing exercise from Martin to bring them to life.

1. **Lean back** so you're not using the muscles of your trunk to support you.
2. **Pick up an object**, any object; it doesn't matter what it is. Bring it to your lap, and using just your hands, explore and notice every detail of that object. Is it pointy? Is it smooth? Rough? Heavy? Light? *Receive the sensations that the object offers to your hands.* Don't worry if your mind wanders, just bring your awareness back to your hands and what they're feeling. Go slowly—Martin describes, "slowing your hands down enough to find out what feels interesting, or what feels pleasant." Continue to focus on feeling, reeling in the mind again and again.
3. **Now go *even slower*,** at about half the pace your hands were feeling before, while staying in tune with the sensations your feeling explorations bring. Eventually, all those sensations will begin to feel quite pleasant, and the longer you stay noticing those feelings, the more it will start to feel *really* good. With nothing to take your attention from those good feelings, feeling good becomes all you feel.

4. Feel the click. This focus on the sensations of your hands can create a physiological shift, where your muscles soften, your breath slows, and your brain settles. For some, this is an easy state to achieve, for others, it takes a bit. Don't be surprised if emotions rise to the surface while you're immersed in the sensations of your hands, from relief to confusion, sadness, shame, guilt, even self-doubt.

Stay as long as you like in your feelings and your awareness of your hands. And when you come out of this exercise, remember to feel into your hands a little more often; they carry much more than just car keys and cell phones, and can show you more than you'd think.

From here, let's work together to expand into the areas of pleasure that have previously been blocked by unconscious and reflexive habits. It's important to note that pleasure is not simply sex and orgasm; it is moving energy through an exquisite resonant technology (also known as your body). No matter how far off it may seem, you absolutely can learn how to interact with pleasure, listen to your body, and stop treating yourself the way a domineering and insensitive lover might. Transformation happens one sensual moment at a time. When you serve yourself like your own true love, you serve the world.

RECLAMATION REMEDY: OWN YOUR PLEASURE

PLEASURE HUNT
The pleasure hunt involves (quite literally) the act of following what feels good in the moment, whatever that may be.

First, notice your breath. There are no rules to this practice, no special way to sit or hold your hands to activate the power of this meditation.

Follow your breath and notice sensations in your body. Maybe you want to soften your jaw, relax your throat, or soften your belly.

Go ahead and exaggerate your breath, allowing the jaw to loosen, the throat to open, and the belly to relax.

As you inhale deeply, maybe your chest expands, with collarbones opening and back arching, head tilted back.

As you exhale, collapse forward a bit and drop your head to your chest as your ribs curl in and your tailbone tucks under.

Open and close with your exaggerated breath and string those inhales and exhales together, almost like a rolling fog of breath and motion.

Go bigger with your breath and invite your voice to come out and play. Inhale a long drawn-out gasp, exhale a deep billowing *ahhhh*.

In the midst of this storm of breath, motion, and sound, notice with your brain—*Where is there pleasure here*?

Is there pleasure in the full expression of the inhale, when the lungs are bursting, and your vessel feels ready to explode?

Is there pleasure in the full expression of the exhale, when the lungs feel empty and the calm before the next big breath feels sacred and silent?

Maybe the pleasure was in the process it took to get to the biggest breath, the strongest exhale.

Now it's time to stretch into your breath. As you inhale and exhale, stretch and move in whatever way feels natural, and explore that pleasure.

This is where the hunting part of pleasure hunting begins. As you feel a sensation, you're going to follow it, whether it be in your lower back, your chest, or collar bone; if that inhale makes you aware of a rib that's poking out a bit, move into that sensation.

As you move, feel the movement organically evolve. A stretch to rehome that out of place rib can easily turn into a spiral, as you breathe and sway, stretching forward, to the side, back, then around forward again.

Follow what feels good in the moment and notice all the ways your body plays with the movement. Notice the curves of your body: the strong curve of your jaw or shoulder or the swell of your breasts or belly. Just tune into those curves and pay attention to their feedback.

What is it to move through the world in your wonderfully curved feminine body?

These essentially feminine shapes, pushed into a linear world full of "no" energy—no, don't do that, you shouldn't say that, stay in your lane.

Don't suppress the soft curves; instead play with them and *within* them.

Now, start to invite your sexual energy, your vital force energy, your eros, to come out and play. Invite it into this pleasure hunting experience and explore it without feelings of shame or judgment.

For me, that looks like running my hands over my body, from my legs, up my sides, over my breasts, all while deeply breathing and moving where the pleasure takes me, swaying and spiraling as I sink into my sitz bones and stretch into my chest.

What is it to invite this sexual energy into your experience, unapologetically? Are you ready for it? What does it even mean to you? Where do you feel it in your body?

Does it move up and down your spine? Do you feel it pulsing in your pussy? Does it feel alive in your fingers?

I don't know about you, but so much of my inner sexy shows up in my hair. I want to pull it, tug it, run my fingers through it, massage its roots and mess it up beyond recognition.

Where does this sexual energy live in your body, and can you feel it as you're simply breathing?

Notice it and pay attention to it like you're your very own adoring, devoted partner, as if you're walking through the world your entire life, playing this game with the most extraordinary lover you've ever imagined possible, totally tuned into you.

How would you move if that was your life?

Pretty powerful stuff, right? Amazing, you've just tapped into your inner goddess through pleasure hunting.

Now take your hands and squeeze your arms, giving yourself a big, strong hug, and open your eyes.

Welcome back, beautiful soul. How was the hunting?

TAKING AND RECEIVING PLEASURE

This is an adaptation of another home play assignment from my coach Whitney, where we gently ask the body what it wants and honor it by freely giving it.

Lie down and focus on a feeling of relaxation and safety.

Become aware of where your body presses into the floor or bed. Breathe into the back of your body, your legs, your feet.

When your attention has settled into your body and you feel connected to its needs, ask yourself: "Body, what touch would feel good to you right now?"

Explore your body and look for the touch that resonates best with what your body is craving right now. Maybe it's long, deep strokes down the arms and thighs. Maybe it's a gentle squeeze to the shoulders and neck. It could even be some playfully light scratches up your sides and over your breasts.

Find the touch you want and be present to that touch for at least three breaths. Get it to a delicious place, before you get to overload, and then recenter in the afterglow, just breathing without touch.

Once you feel settled, ask your body again "What would feel good to you now?"

Have fun exploring what your body wants to feel, and give yourself a few breaths to play in. It's possible your body doesn't want any of it and wants a nap or a snack or movement instead. Honor what comes up and don't force anything.

You might even want to have some sensation play props for this exercise. Furs, feathers, crystal dildos, weighted blankets, and even a good old hot water bottle can feel amazing when introduced in a mindful body practice like this.

When you're finished, take a few deep breaths and thank your body for being open to this play session.

Uncovering Your Erotic Blueprint

How would you define good sex?

Both people climaxing, hopefully simultaneously, panting, sweaty, and cuddling afterward?

It turns out that accepting, taking, serving, and allowing—unlocking mutual pleasure—is so much easier when you speak the same language, but we've been raised with different dialects talking *at* each other most of our lives.

Studying the Erotic Blueprints, created by Jaiya, has validated long-held desires and resolved confusion and shame around my own erotic preferences by offering a map for self-exploration and deeper understanding. Like the love languages for sexuality, the Erotic Blueprints categorize parameters of arousal in a way that can be translated to partners to optimize communication and mutual pleasure. While there are as many erotic signatures as people, there are styles that are readily identifiable, and it turns out that there are five kinds of sexy in the human species.[6] Like any relational skill, however, you must know yourself, and the Blueprints are, chiefly, an introduction to your own erotic nature.

Are you turned on by a swift hair pull or would you rather a trail of roses?

Is flogging and bondage a big yes or do you want warm hands hovering inches over your body?

Do you need the perfect temperature, music, and lighting, or is a bathroom stall just fine?

In taking the Erotic Blueprints quiz, I discovered that my primary Blueprint is the "Shapeshifter," which was incredibly validating given how much I've wrestled with the "I'm too much" story in and out of the bedroom. One of my girlfriends wept when she learned she was a Sexual Blueprint, having slut-shamed herself for years; she never knew that for Sexuals, having sex is as essential as drinking water. Another friend, an Energetic, finally understood why she hated when her partner (a Sexual) would take her too quickly. And yet another friend, a Kink-psychological type, understood why power play takes her from zero to sixty in seconds and eye gazing as foreplay made her want to take a nap. With insight into each other's turn-ons, you and your partner can learn what giving really looks like rather than mind reading, guessing, or assuming that he wants the same things you do. And in your self-led erotica, you can begin to honor your erotic energy and take your preferences, sensitivities, and shadows seriously.

212

EROTIC BLUEPRINTS

Energetic

If you've ever discovered (or suspected) that you can orgasm without being touched, you might be Energetic. Aroused by the Big Tease, a hypersensitive Energetic can be overwhelmed if attention is too direct or intense, so keep it light and play with joyful anticipation. You might be more intuitive than some, and your sexual connections are usually much more than skin deep. To be able to fully surrender to the erotic energy, safety is key for turn-on, and grounding breathwork can help to keep your head in the game. Without the right environment, Energetics can feel overwhelmed and anxious, and can often clam up when things get too hot and heavy too soon. Slow down, enjoy the anticipation, and ease into contact.

Sensual
Ambiance is key for the Sensual, because fully engaging all senses is your recipe for success. You'll find yourself aroused by the right surroundings that activate sight, smell, taste, touch, and sound. On the other hand, anything jarring or out of place can pull you out of sexy time and land you right in your head, which is an erotic roadblock to avoid, especially for Sensuals. Sensation play can be an infinite reservoir, and there's a whole tickle trunk of exercises and props to help you explore all your delightful senses. Blindfolds, ice cubes, and candles—Oh my! Every sense is a portal to pleasure for Sensuals, who tend to love deeper, firmer touch and contact. Set the container right with temperature, scent, lighting, music, and soft fuzzy blankets and watch the pleasure unfurl.

213

Sexual
Sex is your superpower and your supercharger. You approach sex with a sense of playful fun, and orgasm is your grand prize. You don't need to make a production of it, so while others might need a well-lit love nest and a stack of poetry filled letters to get excited, you just need hot, driving, visceral (usually penetrative) sex to get your juices flowing. Of note: your intense focus on frequent genital-based pleasure and penetrative sex can sometimes make relationships difficult with partners who don't share your sex-centric blueprint.

Kinky
Are you titillated by the taboo side of sexual exploration? If you're drawn to power dynamics, fetish-based scenes, restraint and impact toys, and challenging sexual norms ... congratulations, you're probably quite Kinky. But society likes to shame the things you love, and it can take

some work to undo all that programming to really let your freak flag fly proud! With both psychological and physical subtypes, kink is about the use of delineated roles and often employs tools for bondage, sensation, and impact to create the portal through which a couple can walk into transcendent erotic states.

Shapeshifter

Much like a kid in a candy store, the Shapeshifter wants it all and won't be happy until they've tried everything! Fresh, new, and exciting experiences are essential to your arousal, so it's important for you to have a partner who's willing to explore with you. You probably already have a pretty robust sexual tool kit, with toys to cater to any whim and fulfill any fantasy, and your bucket list of sexual desires is most likely an ambitious one. Shapeshifters can sometimes feel like their sexual interests and needs are "too much," however, when fully embraced, Shapeshifter types can tap into any Blueprint style that the moment calls for and feel inspired and resourced.

214

CHAPTER 14

Living the Reclaimed Life

By now you've waded through the Big *No* and Hell *Yes* of your initia-tory journey. You've had your rupture of individuation and you are operating more from Your Self, you amazing self-initiate, you! What follows in this chapter are my key tips, tricks, and takeaways for the Reclaimed Woman to dance through life with delight—or at the *very* least move toward far more fulfilling experiences in the potentially stickiest realms of relationship, mothering, and entrepreneurship.

Get ready to see how to apply the Reclaimed Woman principles to every aspect of your life. We'll begin with reclaimed relationships, because the love affair inside you will be reflected in the love affairs outside.

Reclaimed Woman Relationships

WHY WE PICK THE WRONG PEOPLE
OVER AND OVER AGAIN

"When someone shows you who they are, believe them the first time."

—*Maya Angelou*

We might like to think that we choose partners based on a personal checklist of values, attributes, and characteristics, in a meaningfully arranged hierarchy of importance. Unfortunately, this framework does not account for the quite powerful (*and unconscious!*) dimensions of attraction and partnering. As we explored in Part 1, we learned what love is from our caregivers, and because many of us were loved conditionally, we learned which of our behaviors resulted in connection and which resulted in withdrawal of parental affection, approval, and warmth, or worse, resulted in violence. This outward-focused survival strategy (often aggrandized as empathy) threatens our connection to our feelings, intuition, and even our own minds.

In the crucible of these hot and cold dynamics, we studied our parents so that we could read and anticipate what would keep them appeased, and you likely did not experience the nurturing of your intuitive compass. Instead of the unfoldment of your unique, boundaried personhood—your emergent Self-ness—you adopted intergenerational programs, beliefs, and ideas without any room to question them. And this is why we find ourselves, as a human collective, struggling with the consequences of an unquestioning, obedient, compliant, fear-based populace relating destructively to parentified Mommy Medicine and Daddy Government.

Conditioning keeps us dancing, anticipating, and guessing what our loved one wants and needs so that we can fulfill, appease, and manage expectations to keep the peace. If love felt like chasing, if it felt like we got a crumb for good performance and that negative attention was better than none, then it's no wonder that the same can feel like home in a partner. This power dynamic stems from the sense that someone more powerful dictates our access to feelings of safety, wellbeing, and warmth: what we know as love.

Harville and Helen Hendrix, founders of Imago Therapy, posit that relationships and marriages result from needs rather than love, since our subconscious image of familial love guides our attraction to a partner. This partner will have the same injurious traits as one or both of our parents, and the pairing will then be an opportunity to heal and transform that childhood pain, resolving this pattern of abandonment, rejection, or betrayal. They further theorize that romantic conflict invites these hurts to be felt, and ultimately

healed, chiefly through our own ability to learn to now love ourselves. Because these partners will have complementary wounds, they
will be literally unable to give us what we long for, and we, in turn,
will be unable to give them what they long for.

When we attempt to meet our needs without either overtly declar-
ing them or assessing the potential for them to be met by a given
partner, we default to old strategies of securing needs indirectly:
through manipulation. For example, if you feel jealousy but don't
think your partner will be able to hold, honor, and respond to that
feeling in you, you might criticize or malign a woman you imagine
he would be attracted to. You might insist that you know better than
your partner what he needs to do to succeed, heal, or progress in life,
attempting to control and fix him so that he might one day show
you the love that you want (cue the Rescuer entry point to the victim triangle). Or maybe you want to feel supported, so you develop
a chronic illness that will justify the attention and help that you're
seeking. Or you might say things like, "No woman would ever put
up with this!" Because you don't feel like you can say, "This hurts,
and it doesn't work for me."

When we are disconnected from an awareness of our own needs,
these dynamics can often be described as codependent, and our
needs continue to go largely unmet as we focus on the management
of our partner's expectations, driven by a deep fear of abandonment
and rejection. Codependence stems from a conditioned deficiency
of self-love and results in poor boundaries, poor self-awareness, and
a compromised connection to our needs and how to represent them
with maturity.

The most identifiable marker of codependence is resentment: the
blame of others for one's own self-betrayal. We try to mind read,
to assess stability, and assume we will earn points for all our "loving behavior." We please, often in violation of our own desires. This
works until it doesn't. Then we play the martyr card that says, "After
all I've done for you . . . you treat me like this?!" In codependent
dynamics, we are unable to actually see, accept, and allow the person

217

to first be who they are, and then decide whether or not we would still choose the relationship. Instead, we hold this partner up against an overlay. We manipulate, judge, and expect them to match our projections. This dynamic is predicated on attachment to a partner's unlived potential, a fantasy, while rejecting who they have shown us they are. This is not love. In this model of "love," everything is on a ledger. It's a transaction. It's a kind of love that keeps score and is ultimately between energetic opponents that are negotiating their way through a seemingly endless minefield of childhood hurt.

Attachment Styles & Whom You Choose

In *Facing Love Addiction*, Pia Mellody describes the common pairing of Love Addicts with Love Avoidants.
She describes Addicts as:
1. Assigning a disproportionate amount of time, attention, and "value above themselves" to the person to whom they are addicted.
2. Having unrealistic expectations for positive regard from the other person in the relationship.
3. Neglecting to care for or value themselves while they are in the relationship.

Avoidants, on the other hand:
1. Evade intensity within the relationship by creating intensity in activities (usually addictions) outside the relationship.
2. Avoid being known in the relationship in order to protect themselves from engulfment and control by the other person.
3. Avoid intimate contact with their partners, using a variety of processes called "distancing techniques."[1]

Love Addicts become neurochemically, behaviorally, and psychologically addicted and conditioned around cycles of positive and negative intensity, experiencing this as "passion." They are seeking the knight (or maiden) in shining armor who will finally resolve the pain of their original childhood abandonment, betrayal, or rejection experience, but they find the frog or the beast that needs to be somehow magically loved into the prince or king.

Although Addicts are typically the female partner and Avoidants the male, each can be either and even shapeshift between them. Because Love Addicts believe they want connection and closeness, but subconsciously actually fear intimacy, they will do something to create distance from their partner when closeness presents itself. What they actually seek is enmeshment or the childlike merger with an idealized parental figure. As the Addict seeks enmeshment and to source energy from the Avoidant, the Avoidant re-experiences the fear of engulfment from the enmeshment trauma of their own childhood, and is, in response, hypersensitive to being controlled. Thus, they create distance.

Over the course of the relationship, the Avoidant will put up walls of silence and anger (instead of healthy boundaries that facilitate intimacy) to distance from the Addict and minimize intensity within the relationship while seeking increasing stimulus (work, sex, substances) outside of the relationship.

Next comes the rupture of idealization. This rupture and the associated cognitive dissonance (if he loved me this would not be happening) can present an opportunity. At this fork in the road, and certainly through the Imago framework, one partner's sensitivity can serve as a path to healing the other partner's primary defenses. If my household was very volatile growing up, I might long for a calm, rational partner who has the same defensive structure as I do. But in an Imago match or co-addicted dynamic, my partner has the same volatility patterns as my parents, whose patterns developed as they adapted to their own wounding, and my calm rationality might be exactly what they don't want.

This funhouse of reflected, largely impersonal, behavioral patterns ends up feeling hyper-personal and when poorly navigated, can be the death knell of these dynamics. What begins with efforts to please each other devolves into a zero-sum power struggle. This rupture may represent an opportunity for one or both partners to individuate from the relationship (a.k.a. break up), or for the projections and overlays to resolve, and for each partner to truly see the person in front of them for who they've likely always shown themselves to be. In Imago dynamics that last long-term, the partners grow and change in ways that meet each other's needs and serve each person's experience of growing self-love.

For the Love Addict, this kind of breakup can feel as if it requires an inpatient rehab. For the Avoidant, however, because they were not actually in the relationship in the same way but derived a sense of worth from caretaking, serving, and rescuing, the breakup is a very different process that may flare subconscious abandonment wounds leading to an amplification of existing addictions (work, substances, or sourcing attention from other individuals).

Leaving these relationships, the Avoidant and Addict may still go on to repeat the cycle with a new partner. It may, however, be the opportunity of a lifetime to individuate, integrate, and heal, self-sourcing validation, soothing, approval, care, and love in order to attract partners that can offer (and receive) healthy love.

There is a paradox at the very center of love. It is the primacy of *self*-allegiance, *self*-loyalty, and *self*-alignment which opens the heart to pour a superfluity of compassion, approval, and warmth into another no matter what they do, don't do, are, or aren't. This view recognizes that loving does not cost us anything, is non-transactional, and unattached, as long as we are the keepers of our own hearts, narratives, and clear boundaries. If I've got me, and I know what I need, what works for me, and what doesn't, then my choices are what keep me safe, and my embodied feelings will show me where to buy eggs and where to buy hammers.

220

RECLAMATION REMEDY: BREAKUP BREAKTHROUGH

Here is a general framework for navigating the heartbreak of a relationship's ending and giving yourself permission to be a wholly feeling being while you come back to yourself.

If you are entering the dark night of the soul that ending a challenging relationship can represent, remember the big lie we always tell ourselves: that it will feel like this forever.

Remember that change is the only constant.

Take it hour by hour. Maybe half an hour by half an hour. Maybe one breath at a time. Make space to allow for the mess, the confusion, the disorientation. Remember, this is the chrysalis phase. This is precisely *how* you move through the childhood terror of love lost into the emancipation of attracting the safe, fulfilling, stable adult love that does indeed await you.

Stay in your lane

Enter through the upset as many times as it takes. Stay with your own felt experience. Scream, dance, punch, vent, cry. When you feel the shocks of withdrawal, sit down, put your own hand on your own heart and track the sensation inside. Tell your roiling emotions, I'm here with you. I'm not going anywhere. Then WAIT until the sensation transforms. Be with yourself. When your attention flies into his world, his reasoning, dissecting his motives, gently return your attention to you, like a walking meditation through your sovereign life.

It's not your job to educate him

It's so tempting to be the one who explains what's going on, why he's messed everything up, and how it could have been better. If you were skilled at mutual repair, you'd still be together, however, so odds are the communication channels have some blocks and the defenses have some serious incompatibilities. If he doesn't ask for your perspective and you attempt to educate him, the impulse likely derives from the sense that "getting him to see" will bring you safety. The intention to correct another's understanding is a sign of self-abandonment and an opportunity to get back into your lane.

There he is again

He has already shown you who he is, perhaps from the first interaction. To feel indignation, resentment, shock, or disturbance around a more recent display of this familiar behavior is to remain in a kink. So, there he is again! Unattuned, irrational, volatile, or defensive ... there he is, being the person he's always shown himself to be. Nothing new to report here. Nothing to see. Back to your lane!

Resolve superiority

The mirror is never more operative than in romantic relationships, and if you're triggered by his post-relationship behavior, the mirror is still shining. How is it that you could be doing exactly what you imagine he is doing to you? Are you expecting an irrational person to be rational? Isn't that irrational? Are you only interested in your own perspective, judging him for his narcissism? Are you lying to yourself about what you've always known in your bones to be true about him while calling him a liar? Ask yourself if you are doing the same to him or to yourself that you're accusing him of doing. Get to the place where you can truly say, I am not superior to him. Because you're not. I'm not. No one is.

Alchemize resentment into needs

When you think about your former partner, what is it that you tolerated in the relationship? How have you been hurt? What was your biggest struggle? Underneath these complaints is a desire. If my partner never asked me how I felt and I hated that, then I know that I want to be asked how I feel. If I hated my partner's flirtatious nature, then I long for attention. How does emotional connection, loyalty, and safety actually look for you? What is it that you now understand that you need?

Give up all hope

Explore the possibility that your former partner will *never* be who you wished and wanted and hoped they could be. When we are projecting our parents onto partners, we are little children longing for that primal love. Of course, everyone has hope for healing, and anything is possible, but when you leave a relationship, you are saying, I release you to your destiny, whatever that might look like. When you can let go of the fantasy, you will experience the grief of that original lost love and it may feel like a decimating tidal wave. Let it flow.

Thank you and bye-bye

Journal, furiously or giddily, cathartically about:

- All the things you will NEVER DEAL WITH AGAIN because you are leaving this relationship. Celebrate that liberation!
- Everything that you appreciated about your partner so that you don't continue to erotically caress the enemy. How did he show you love and treat you right? How can you sense his good intent? What was right about the relationship?
- What your partner rejected about you and all the ways you are getting to know, love, and accept these things about yourself (seeing the truth in triggering judgment).
- Why it needed to be exactly this way for you to learn to love yourself that much more. How was he the perfect catalyst?

Create a ritual offering

Light a candle, put on a song you both loved and write a Ho'oponopono prayer:

223

I'm sorry,
Please forgive me,
Thank you,
I love you.

My friend Akasha shared that the Hawaiian prayer traditionally only consisted of "Thank you" and "I love you." This abridged version resonates with what I've learned from Family Constellations, which is that forgiveness is often offered from a place of superiority. If it helps to move old stories onto the page, include "I'm sorry" and "Please forgive me." Otherwise, you can simply offer "Thank you" and "I love you" to the page, in honor of your shared experience, and release that to the ether.

Make art

Write a poem, make a skit, paint a painting, sing a song, dance a dance that would be written, painted, sung, played, or moved from the part of you that is feeling the most intensely. What does that part want to share with the world? Or just your loving witness consciousness? Consider how you can truly embody the character that feels forsaken, betrayed, misunderstood, or violated and create from that place. Offer it to the collective or make it just because art wants to be made.

Know that every relationship, every heartbreak, every repeat of an old pattern is here because we need it to be exactly this way. Let us embrace what is. When we are ready for the expansion that is our birthright, we will move with courage through the lies our sweet minds tell us (just trying to keep us safe!), through the fear that clenches our hearts, and we will quickly taste the liberation, the inner okayness, and even the wonder at the unexpected delight of receiving exactly what we've always wanted when and where we may least expect it.

You've got this.

RECLAMATION REMEDY: LEARNING TO LOVE

Choice is the path of reclamation, and awareness of needs is what generates choice. We all have unfinished business from childhood: experiences that were overwhelming to our tiny nervous systems—too much, too soon, too fast—and flagged as dangerous. These traumatic experiences can range from a harsh look from a math teacher all the way through to incest and violence, and they were given instantaneous meaning by us as children. Since those feelings of fear, shame, and grief became associated with near death-level risk, we recruit behavioral strategies such as appeasement, withdrawal, defensiveness, and manipulation to keep from ever feeling those feelings again, stuffing decades-old emotions beneath the floorboards. We made these experiences mean that we are unlovable, broken, unworthy, and worse, often remain in idealized Stockholm Syndrome defense of our caregivers' "best intentions."

As adults, life delivers us relational patterns of conflict, upset, and unfulfillment so that we can complete our childhood experiences and offer our child-self the love, attention, presence, and validation that was not available back when we needed them the most. These patterns are here to invite that exiled part of us that is holding all those feelings back home.

Let's take a deep dive into identifying your top three relational needs, which primarily surface in romantic relationships, but are often just as present in platonic and familial dynamics.

There are four steps that are to be engaged at your own pace:

1. Reflect on your most memorable grievances in your recent adult life. What are the things you

225

resent the most or that have made you most upset? For example: I resent that I always "have to" plan the dates with my husband. I resent that my wife always says she's going to come home in ten minutes, and she comes home in thirty. I resent that I feel punished for having a different opinion than my sister. I resent that my friend always talks about herself and never asks me how I feel.

2. Resentment is a sign of a need being unmet. The twist is that it's YOU who abandoned, betrayed, or rejected yourself, and that is now being experienced as someone else doing that to you. So look at your resentment list and write down what you would have liked to have happen in that instance instead. Literally. For example: I want my husband to initiate plans. I want my wife to stick to her word. I want my sister to be open and curious and stay connected even if I have a different idea than her. I want my friend to care about me enough to ask how I feel.

3. Now we're going to the root; the list of prompts on the next page is a serious endeavor. Clear about an hour, make yourself comfortable, and then do something to make yourself even a little more comfortable, and then answer as many questions as you can as if you were writing honestly to your mother and then to your father. Don't overthink it; let it flow. Handwritten is best.

   Do you see any themes emerging between your adult needs and those that came through in journaling about your parents? Can you see how you've chosen partners just like your parents? What about you? Have you taken on traits just like your mom or dad even though the same traits were hurtful to you as a child?

4. Based on the above, choose three emotional needs that summarize what you most want (that you didn't get and often don't get in your adult relationships).

Share these needs with your partner, or just a friend, and find one way that you can start to offer yourself the experience of meeting your needs. For example:

- If validation is a big one for you, offer yourself approval.
- If being respected is important to you, monitor your internal dialogue for disrespectful self-talk.
- If another's integrity matters to you, honor your own word.

Answer these prompts as if you were writing about yourself to your mother and then your father:

- The three most challenging aspects about you are . . .
- My most painful memory is . . .
- I would feel scared of you when . . .
- You often told me I should/shouldn't . . .
- What I needed from you that I didn't receive . . .
- If you were to describe me, you would say . . .
- The way I knew you loved me was . . .
- The easiest way to feel connected to you was . . .
- My three favorite qualities about you are . . .
- My most prized memory is . . .
- I feel/felt safe with you when . . .
- Your relationship to my mother/father taught me . . .
- Your relationship to money taught me . . .
- Your relationship to sex/sexuality taught me . . .
- Your relationship to work and success taught me . . .
- Your relationship to health taught me . . .
- My most recent memory of a painful interaction was . . .
- I am still angry with you because . . .

- When I think of you today, I feel . . .
- I'd like to tell you this about myself . . .
- I forgive you for . . .
- Thank you for teaching me how to . . .

You cannot experience emotional security by un-needing your needs; emotional security requires the direct meeting of these needs. The good news is that you can ask for your needs to be met in your current relationships, and you can also begin to meet your own needs. This awareness is game-changing, and it is the beginning of developing self-trust, loyalty, and love so that you can actually attract, receive, and experience another person's love and presence in a way that your child self never knew possible.

SURRENDER TO HIS DEPTH
An adaptation of an exercise from David Deida

If you're a strong, capable woman, you might find dating very difficult. If you've ever heard the words "You're amazing, you're wonderful, *but* I know I can't give you what you want—I'm not good enough for you," then you might be choosing the wrong men to try to build something lasting with. You repeatedly choose men you do not fully respect, trust, and who do not inspire surrender. From that place of felt superiority, you know that you can always be in control, always depend on yourself, and always be "safe." At some point, your heart's yearning becomes irrepressible, and you long to feel led by the man you choose. How do you attract the type of man that you can truly surrender to?

First, get super clear on the man you want. Usually, the kind of man you can fully surrender to is emotionally self-regulated, self-realized in his purpose, and he is, in a word, *deep*. A deep man is one whom you can trust to guide you *spiritually*. This doesn't mean that he does more meditation, plant medicine, or yoga than you. It means that you trust him to lead you in ways that you cannot lead yourself, to know the next best step better than you do, and to hold your heart with devotional care.

As David Deida puts it in his signature fashion, walk the world with your head high, your shoulders back, and energetically offer to the men you encounter, "Take me, I'm yours, and if you're shallow, I'll kill you. Take me, I'm yours, and if you can't meet me where I am, I'll kill you."

Now, nobody is getting murdered, but rejection can feel a little bit like death when the heart is involved, so be as melodramatic as you like with your phrasing. The gist of the sentiment should set a strong intention for the kind of partner you're looking for. Try out:

"If you aren't my spiritual equal (or superior), please do not apply."
"If you can't lead me to new realizations and new paradigms of evolution, I ask you to kindly fuck right off."
"If you are what I need you to be, and can live up to your promise, I'll follow you anywhere."
"If I can't surrender to your depth, don't waste my time."[2]

Watch how these phrases allow for that soft heart and strong spine to take shape so that you can more accurately perceive with the divining rod of your body, who can take you deeper.

Become the Surrendered Wife

Even if you say you want a strong man, you may need help aligning your behavior to become the wife who invites her husband to serve, protect, provide, and caretake your heart, needs, and pleasure. Brimming with utterly life-changing gems and reframes, *The Surrendered Wife* by Laura Doyle will not fit through the sieve of your feminist programming, so I'm glad we've moved on. Claiming to have fixed over fifteen thousand marriages, Doyle asserts that women can learn intimacy skills to transform marriages that would otherwise be left for dead. There's no "toxic" dynamic too problematic for Doyle, who believes that women have the power to transform neglect, infidelity, and even abuse: no couples counseling required. In fact, your husband doesn't need to read her book, go to a therapist, do plant medicine, or follow a guru. It's you, woman, who has the power to change the dynamic.

For example, one of her revolutionary tips is affectionately referred to as "duct tape." Simply put, *shut up* more often. The next time your husband is driving, pay close attention to your need to micromanage his speed, his direction, and his choices. This is more than a metaphor; this is a literal barometer for how much you are willing to trust and respect the man that you have chosen. Secure that figurative duct tape over your mouth and just don't say anything about his driving . . . for the whole ride. Nada. And then take that practice home. Whenever you have the urge to "help out" your man, that's the perfect moment to pipe down. Reminder, your inner victim lives in your "helper," and so does the mommy-son dynamic that buries even the most erotic partnerships under heavy piles of trauma. Whenever you imagine that you can "man better than your man," or figure it all out for him, it's a surefire sign that it's time to quit talking and get back in your lane, focused on you.

A husband needs to learn from *life*, Doyle says, not his *wife*, and that "helpful" in wife language means "critical" in husband language. Doyle stresses the importance of allowing your husband to manage the finances and providership and letting him fail as you resist the urge to do for him what he can do for himself and for you. When a man asks for your advice, the temptation to put your mom jeans on and show him the way can feel irresistible. You likely find yourself getting a hit of significance, value, and worth, but before you know it, you're well on your way to a polarity disaster. So, what if in those moments you could meet him with these simple words: "That's a great question. What do *you* think you should do?" Shifting the conversation back to him sends the message that you totally, wholeheartedly trust your man's judgment. It confers a sense of *I know you got this, and I'm just going to sit here in admiration as you figure it out.*

A husband requires trust and respect if he is to provide you with presence, attention, and protection. It's that simple; if you want to be in the wife archetype, start by treating your man (the one you chose and for good reason) as though he's a man worth respecting. Ditch the advising, the micromanaging, and the overall control tactics that are only working against you. Quit taking the bait of petty, naggy litigations and remain focused inward. When your focus is within, you'll be able to identify what you want and to ask for it with pure desire. He is designed to solve the problem of you not having what you want, especially when your desire isn't framed as his deficiency.

As a woman, surrendering to a man isn't about resigning or giving up anything; it's not about being controlled. It's about creating the conditions for the containment you seek.

RECLAMATION REMEDY:
IMPROVE YOUR RELATING WITH MEN RIGHT NOW

Become a surrendered wife like Laura Doyle
In short, you can have control or you can have intimacy. Releasing control means that you assess the rightness of a given situation, relationship, or circumstance for you, you source okayness within, and you offer your open

---

heart, knowing it feeds you to do so. Next time you feel like you're tightening the grip with your man, try one of these reframes:

- Ask your man for help, giving him an opportunity to feel needed and useful.
- When he inquires about what to do, let go of the wheel and say, specifically, "Whatever you think."
- Rather than nagging him for his lack of attention, simply say, "I miss you . . . "
- Let him fail without criticism and nagging. Choose to trust him and support him in his role.
- Know what you want and ask for it with "I'd love . . . "
- Don't do for your partner what they are capable of doing themselves just because you imagine you can do everything better or faster.
- Receive what is given or gifted with gratitude.
- Own it (and apologize) when you are disrespectful.
- Focus on your own happiness, fulfillment, and pleasure, every day.[3]

When we reclaim this power, take responsibility for our own inner healing, and begin to learn how to relate with intention instead of taking the bait, suddenly our need to blame, criticize, and reduce men falls away. Instead, we start to enjoy genuinely appreciating men who are behaving with integrity, supporting us, or otherwise trying their best.

Relationship Repair Resources:
Reveal
When something feels out of integrity, express it as wordlessly as possible with "oof" or "that hurts," and watch your man rise to solve the problem of your pain.

Stay in your lane
If his behavior is confronting some tender spots in you, rather than let him know what he's doing wrong, stay focused on your feelings, and then go to him with a pure desire "I'd love" ask.

Don't criticize his actions
Celebrate when he's getting it right (also a great parenting tip). Look into his eyes and tell him: I feel safe with you when you do that. It feels so good. Exaggerate and amplify this enthusiasm for the people in the back.

Create containers
Don't talk about everything all the time. Ask consent and set a timer! Say, "I'd like to talk about what's coming up for me for fifteen minutes at 5 p.m. Does that work?" This is also an epic strategy for the working woman who may need help transitioning from girl-bossing to a surrendered wife. Take one hour to get yourself into your body with a bath, music, a quick full body shake, self-massage, or aromas so that you stay in the pleasure of being an embodied woman offering your man your soft open heart, respect, and regard.

Allow space
If you're a recovering anxious attachment girlie, you may feel like your oxygen mask is pulled off when there is a stalemate, or when he seems to need space. Just ask how much space and time he needs and then give it to him!

MAKE EVERY MAN BIGGER
Om Rupani calls this effort "making every man bigger," an essential intention for restoring the masculine at the helm of society to serve, protect, and provide for the feminine.

Om says that men have a green light and a red light, so learn how to press the green for the good of all. Express authentic appreciation, from your heart, every time you notice a man (friend, lover, or stranger) making your life better.

Don't speak ill of them

Make a commitment with your girlfriends to no longer shit-talk men, which includes generalizations or complaining about your partner (or exes). I've let all my partnered friends know that I am no longer available to collude in making men wrong. This means that I'm not taking her side; I'm not circling around the drain with stories of his bad behavior, and I'm not playing the Rescuer to the victim she is in her relationship. It's not easy to resist the bait, but I choose to live in a world where romance is no longer a zero-sum game. Plus, do you really want to be a woman who is surrounded by men who mistreat her, or a woman who's had a million toxic exes? Be the queen and honor the man at your side, and the men of your past.

Don't waste a man's attention

If a man's superpower is his attention, do you really want to waste this precious resource by chatting about what's happening on your favorite Netflix show and the latest annoying thing your girlfriend did? Honor your man's attention, choose your time and activities together with discretion, and remember that your girlfriends are there for chitty chat.

Guard his reputation

If a man's honor is as valuable to him as his life, then how would you protect and serve that? It would start with never speaking disrespectfully of him to others, in front of others, and regarding his privacy and integrity as precious.

Reminder: You don't surrender to him for *him*. You surrender to him because you chose him as the channel of consciousness, and you know that, when you do, he can take you to places you simply cannot go on your own.

Real Love & Choosing Your Partner

Healthy attachment, or the formation of loving and secure bonds in relationships, offers us a safe haven from the perils of life, and the benefits of emotional co-regulation have been documented in multiple studies. For example, in a groundbreaking functional MRI study, brain scans showed how a woman can be offered containment by a man who intentionally provides loving touch. The study begins by placing the woman in an MRI, where she is subjected to a threat cue (an ankle shock), and her brain responses were recorded as her partner held her hand. Then, after the couple attended months of Emotionally Focused Therapy (EFT), an approach that seeks to repair adult attachment bonds, the woman went back into the scanner to be re-exposed to threat cues while her partner held her hand. Amazingly, the EFT-mediated establishment of more secure attachments enabled women to experience less pain and anxiety the second time around, as their partners were able to provide nervous system co-regulation.[4] I believe that we ALL need a model for healthy masculine-feminine polarity; most of us never had one, and very few of us know where to find it.

So, once you've freed yourself up to choose differently, how do you actually choose a partner who is a match for the healthy dyad that polarity work suggests is fully available to us?

Through family constellations, I've come to know that there are three *Yes's* of true love, proffered by constellations therapist Marine Sélénée in her excellent book, *Connected Fates, Separate Destinies*. These *Yes's* would indicate that you're a full-body *Yes* to dive into the depths of true intimacy with your potential partner. Anything less than the following should warrant serious reconsideration, as you're likely in the funhouse of projections rather than the I-thou gaze of adult connection.

1. You must be a 100 percent full-body yes to this man *as he is*. No project, no "maybe one day he'll get sober." No shadow

work mandates. If you want to meet your partner in the realm of true intimacy, you've got to accept the person you see in front of you, right now.

2. In just the same way that you must accept the person in front of you, you must accept their parents as an extension of them. You must accept that this person is made from his parents and permanently connected to those beings.

3. Finally, you *must* say yes to this person's separate destiny. If love is contingent upon the relationship itself existing in a certain way, it may not be love.

As someone who is no stranger to trauma bonds, my sense is that the best man for you is the one who allows your system to exhale. And the best woman for a man is the one who inspires him to protect and provide. In other words, healthy chemistry allows a woman to be a woman (and not a mommy!) and a man to be a man. The egregore of marriage and sacred union becomes available through devotion to something that affords each individual a sense of true belonging rather than conditional love and eroticized wounds. And perhaps gatekeeping our sexual energy until commitment is established may actually serve to identify a man's capacity to do what should come most naturally to a mature man: claim you.

Speaking of choosing, let's illuminate my latest sovereign choice that came to be from probing my deepest desires: choosing motherhood.

Reclaimed Woman Mothering
CLAIMING JOY AND CHOOSING MOTHERHOOD

What is sovereign love? I would venture that there is no better dynamic riper for the exploration and expansion of love than the mother-child dyad.

In her book *Conscious Femininity*, Jungian analyst Marianne Woodman illuminated that the maiden, mother, crone triad is better depicted as mother, virgin, crone, wherein the conscious mother makes way for the stage in a woman's lifescape where she is virginal or *unto herself.* The virgin is self-sourcing and has the courage to be and the flexibility to always be *becoming.* In this way, the mother archetype fuses devotional service with self-actualization. Motherhood is the incubator within which we learn intimacy through our children who lead us home to ourselves as virgins and later wise elders.

It is not lost on me that my children ignited my awakening process. In fact, sometimes I think I became a mother semi-consciously because I *knew* in the seat of my soul that they would wake me up from the haze of disembodied disconnection that characterized my life. My self-initiation was delivered to me in the form of natural birth and a postpartum diagnosis of Hashimoto's Thyroiditis, and I was poised for my heroine's journey home. But my *No* phase put me deep into the dark forest, and my meandering led me toward the anonymous victim and away from my home and from my daughters' father.

As we've explored, there have been many bait-and-switch moments in our journey as women collectively and individually, and one of the potential poor bargains that we have made is "I will follow my mission and my purpose. I will prioritize my work, and it won't cost anything because I can still be a mom." No, dear woman, you *cannot* have it all, and work-life balance is as much a figment as the fruits of egalitarian man-mimicking feminism. I was able to hide from my own choice to prioritize my mission and my work because I decided that I "had" to be the breadwinner, and because I have an Italian mama and a devoted father who stepped in to buffer the natural consequences. So, for the first few years of my daughters' lives, I chose to prioritize work, and for the following eight, I chose to prioritize a man who was not their father.

And when I chose to leave this second relationship, my daughters exhaled, and I was delivered my next opportunity to learn how to love: myself and my girls. I began to offer myself the sense of safety that I imagined would come from a partner, from a system, or even from a family system, and to experience the emergent gifts and embodied self-expression that spring forth after that safety is more consistently established. Choosing celibacy, I've focused on my home life, what lights me up, and our pink, feminine, jewel box of a house.

In this process, I have also decided to take on a life of more intentional sobriety. At a certain point, it became clear to me that eliminating all sources of consciousness-altering substances from my life was the path to claiming more of my mystical superpowers. From the outside in, the change may have been imperceptible, but I had, through my choice to go all in on my life without an escape hatch, grown the capacity to hold divergent realities, to wear my Villain Crown, and to allow my girls to be who they each are . . . and not a moment too soon. As they entered their years of individuation as teens, the subtle but powerful enmeshment trauma that I imposed through the *I know better than you what you need for you* approach to holistic mothering was beginning to unravel.

I could see clearly that when I was pushing my truther perspectives on them, informing them about how they should eat, how they should relate to their self-care, or what kinds of bras they should be wearing, there was a deep shadow at play, showing me my own fear.

I was also shown that even though I thought that I was ready for sacred union with a perfect polarity partner, I struggled to envision how this man would blend with my daughters, my animals, and my home. Would I keep my home as a personal investment and move into his with my girls? Would I live half my life with my daughters here and the other with him? But what about my pets? I just couldn't seem to make the vision work . . .

No matter how many times I attempted to convince myself of all the wonderful reasons a beautiful man could add to our lives, I would wrestle with the fear that this was simply not in the cards for me. In my darker moments, I felt forsaken by God. I felt alone and abandoned and deep in the martyr energy of *why do I have to do all of this alone?*

Until a cataclysmic moment in my friend Sarah's kitchen exposed this divided will around partnership and mothering. I have some gorgeous girlfriends, and Sarah is no exception. Five years my senior, she is the age that I will be when my daughters leave the house. Five years, that's all I have left. The notorious teen years where the future foundations for adult intimacy with one's children are established. It's as if we test our parents in these years to determine how emotionally equipped they are to allow us to grow and become, and the result can be seen in the nature of the connection going forward. So, in front of Sarah, I couldn't tell myself that if I waited five years to call in my husband, I'd be a withered menopausal hag, since she is vital, hot, and enjoying her life to the fullest. And, in front of her, I sat in full awareness of the power of choosing motherhood because I watched her do it with her extraordinary kids, both of whom have now emancipated while remaining connected to her. I watched her put her role as mother first, for their entire childhoods, and now I am watching her explore her creativity, pleasure, and passions out in the world while her children call to update her on their life adventures.

239

Sobbing in Sarah's arms, I saw the truth like a thunderclap. I can't make my daughters want a stepdad (does anyone really want a stepdad when they have a fantastic dad?!), and I can't figure out why I've been forsaken. I can't figure it out because it's not meant to be figured out! The truth is that I don't actually *want* a husband now. I want the joy in front of me. I want, before it's too late, to choose to prioritize my role as mother (notice I didn't say prioritize my children, but rather my role and my values). See, my daughters (and their friends) are about as epic as it gets. The belly laughing, inspiration, fun, and pure joy that I experience with them is the highlight of my life. Literally. And it's right in front of me. And I was choosing something that is nowhere to be seen—this imaginary partner—and so deep in that myopic struggle that I might have betrayed myself, again.

In my motherhood journey, I've now landed in the sweet space of pure enjoyment and conscious choice, a place where nothing comes before my priority of mothering which is a natural outgrowth of my prioritization of pleasure and joy . . . my prioritization of self. Not because I feel I should be "that" mom, but because I can't imagine anything I would rather do, and because I am learning to love myself through these angelic teachers. My will is no longer divided, and I am all in, choosing the life that I actually have.

I've reclaimed my own erotic energy from the struggle with what is and the desperation for something that I don't have in the here and now, and the relief is exquisite.

So, what is the joy in front of you that you could choose if you shifted your focus from fixing what's not here to creating with what is?

Victimless Mothering

Waiting in line at a store, my youngest daughter said, "Mama, I love that woman's outfit!" Furrowing my brow, I semi-sarcastically responded, "It's pretty *basic*," clarifying that I, in fact, did *not* love this woman's outfit. That was a solid C-/D on the Mothering report card, and one of many instances of the same.

Why?

Because I did not visit with her reality, and instead, I imposed my own.

On a redo (which you can always claim by way of eventual apology), I might have said, *"Tell me more! What do you like about it?"*

It's so hard to honor our children's sovereignty and to love across different realities. But there is an opportunity here, and it involves learning to hold ourselves emotionally, as adults, in ways that our parents didn't model, owning ourselves so that our children can actually exist as independent beings and not narcissistic extensions vying for conditional attention from us. This is humbling work, but since you've made it this far, I know you're ready for it.

And in the throes of the spiritual and wellness revolution, I also believe it's one of the biggest challenges facing the holistic community: how to not impose rigid beliefs onto our children because we "know better" if they're choosing to eat differently or act differently than we as good wellness warrior mommies want them to.

Take a moment and ask yourself:

Do you believe you have to be your children's savior? That it's your responsibility to completely clear out all your generational trauma so your kids won't have to deal with it? Are you maybe a little bit too invested in being the cycle breaker for your lineage?

Here's another perspective:

What if your children can become an opportunity to learn about yourself, be with yourself, and spiritually mature yourself?

What if they came into this world more actualized and more developed than you give them credit for?

What if your only real work was to hold space for them to be their full Selves and learn about your own full Self along the way?

To that end, here are my top victimless mothering tips, hard won through nearly two decades of inquiry. I would by no means call myself an expert; this work is ongoing, but the more you give to it, even just a little bit of victimless mothering, the more you can bring laughter where there was pain.

RECLAIMED WOMAN VICTIMLESS PARENTING TIPS

1. **Let go of Punishment & Reward.** Alfie Kohn, author of *Unconditional Parenting,* posits that not only punishment (frank abuse, withdrawal of love, time-outs), but also *praise,* can be detrimental to a child's self-development. Imposing "good" and "bad" on behavior and assigning praise and punishment to those behaviors creates a system of rigid control that disconnects a child from intrinsic motivation. Instead, engage in a dynamic of partnership and mutual exploration by openly discussing impulses

---

and *natural* consequences (and no, losing iPad time is not a natural consequence).

2. **Use the phrase "Tell Me More."** Unfortunately, when this is most needed, when emotions are high and your victim consciousness is trying to assert control, this phrase can feel like crunching glass. When your child expresses something you don't agree with, resist the urge to argue your case and invite them to tell you more. Cross the bridge to visit your child's experience because you're the adult and you *can*. For example, if my daughter mentions that she doesn't like sardines, I could say, "That's because your palate is so limited . . . they're good!" or I could say, "What is it you don't like about them?" to build a bridge of connection and togetherness across differences. The *tell-me-more* curiosity is a transmission of "I am here, invested in caretaking your reality. It matters to me. I'm not here to protect and defend mine."

3. **Be ready to apologize.** Relieve and relax the pressure to get it right the first time around. Awareness grows, and there's no statute of limitations around apologies. If one of your parents were able to sincerely apologize for one of your cardinal wounds decades later, it would still heal something deep inside you. I recently went off to create this elaborate trip to Mexico in order to win my girls' attention, and I apologized every single day for some regrettable behavior on my part. It feels good to apologize because it not only models for them that I fuck up sometimes and could not meet my own conditioning in the moment, but also that I'm willing enough to humbly come forward to own my actions.

4. **Resolve the impulse to offer unsolicited criticism or negative feedback.** Recognize that the need to weigh in, unsolicited, comes from fear, and it is rarely helpful. Notice how often you bring forward

highly critical, unsolicited feedback and then dress it up with sayings like, "Oh, I just thought it would help to know." I, myself, have committed to not offering feedback about my children's choices— not about their style, their fashion, their hair, their makeup, their friends, any of it—before asking if my perspective is welcome. I believe it's their choice to adorn, decorate, and celebrate their bodies and to honor their impulses. And when I don't think they should go out in booty shorts, I am growing my capacity to hold uncomfortable feelings as an adult so that my children are not required to manage my inner world. So much "helpful feedback" actually serves to assuage and soothe our emotional immaturity and intolerance as parents. And you don't have to parent that way anymore.

5. **Talk to your children the way you would talk to a friend.** Would you ever snap at a friend in frustration? We speak to our friends in social parameters that we would do well to apply to our children. Ask yourself, *"Would I speak to a friend this way?"*

If you can bear this in mind when you feel the temptation to say things like "Don't make me ask you again!" or "God, your room is always such a mess," you'll feel the restoration of respect and regard that has been drained from the terrain of American parenting. This is about reclaiming the I-thou gaze: that sense of seeing the grandeur and divinity in another, which is only accessible when your heart is open and willing.

6. **Address the shadow of holistic health activism and awareness.** When you wake up to how important your choices are around diet, detox, and consumerism, you can find yourself believing the body is more fragile than you did when you thought it needed pharmaceuticals to survive. And the truth is, the body is energy, and when you bring

fear, dogmatism, and rigidity to the body, it's not better than bringing poison. I'll never forget when my daughter said, *"Mama, you're afraid of so many things!"* while I was on my Joan of Arc high horse, feeling like I was courageously saving her from all the chemicals and radiation there is. When you think you know what's best about everything from gluten-free, natural, sustainable foods, to non-toxic beauty products, and even filtered water, you can create a rigid grid around your children's behavior towards these things. The downside happens when you fail to invite your children into a holistic practice of self-care, informed choices, and reading the language of the body, and set them up to look for approval and acceptance from you instead. It's another facet of the Reward & Punishment dynamic, and it doesn't allow much room for self-sovereignty. Remember what we've learned about taboo energy and recognize that the judgment you extend to your children offers a powerful infusion of energy into exactly that which you judge. As my insightful sage of a daughter, Lucia, once reflected, "Strict parents make sneaky kids!"

7. **Ask these two questions of your children as they grow up.**
Is there anything that I did to upset you that you still feel upset about?

Is there anything that you need from me that I am not giving you?

And then *Listen.* Simply listen, and try not to meet their share with your own version of the story. Show you care and are invested in their perspective and reality. What's so powerful about these two questions is they allow for the lived experience of your children to come forward, in a way that dismantles any false reality you may be living in where you're some kind of savior or hero.

8. **Drop your defenses.** Drop your defensive narrative. If you remember what it was like to be a child, you realize that kids don't care! They aren't concerned with your reasons for what you did; they care about how you made them *feel.* You can cut that emotional abuse cord of defensiveness, and stop that dueling cycle, where you want to be right and plead your narrative. *Just listen.* Immediately, connection becomes available.

9. **Consider the mirror. Recognize that when you are upset by your child, you are probably doing exactly what it is that you're judging in that moment.** When you're demanding respect from your kid, what you're really doing is disrespecting them. When you're insisting that they calm down, you yourself are not calm. This mirror is almost always operative when you're in judgment.

10. **Really truly feel, listen, and sense when they are offering a No of any kind, through their boundary.** I cannot stress this one enough. This means no grabbing, touching, petting your child whenever you damn well feel like it, especially when they've demonstrated that they're really not all that interested in that moment. This means no forcing, coercing, manipulating, or insisting. It's about really sitting on your hands and honoring when your child has displayed some kind of line in the sand. This is how you demonstrate to your children that their *No* holds weight, that their boundaries are important and necessary, and that they are safe to bring them forward to be expressed in a healthy way that will be met and received and therefore honored. Help your child learn the difference between a little no and a little yes inside and only support them through resistance (like going to soccer practice even if he doesn't feel like it) when you're sure there's a little yes in there.

Doesn't it feel good to imagine a world where there's no manipulation, strategy, curation, or mind reading involved in human relationships? Because everyone knows what they need, asks for it, and takes responsibility for their experience? You can create this now.

You can support your children in remaining connected to their inner compass rather than having to reclaim that connection as we are doing now, decades down the line. You can hold space for your children to be the perfect answer to the existential question your lineage has brought forth, and emotional self-mastery is the way to do just that.

Reclaimed Woman Business

I don't believe that women are meant to be breadwinners, single earners, or corporate climbers. I don't believe that our creativity and self-expression is supposed to feel responsible for the car payment and the rent. Unbraiding the native impulse that we each have to create from our survival needs is an essential maturation of the Reclaimed Woman. If you're committed to hustling a job to pay the bills, and don't feel like you have a choice, you do you, but there may come a moment that your soul rattles its cage and whispers, *I'm ready.* And because you're attuned to those impulses and you know that carving out time for superfluous, indulgent, unproductive pleasure is your responsibility, that whisper may turn into an exquisite song. This song can become your business for the sheer delight of magnetizing revenue in exchange for your energy. Female entrepreneurship is a path that can be walked in heels or in combat boots, and I've done both. Trust me, the stilettos are way more fun. . .

246

Reclaimed Woman Money Matters

Masculine money

This is what I refer to as "functional money." It's the money that pays your damn bills and puts a roof over your head: your groceries, rent, car payments, and everyday essentials. This is the money that's operationalized and distributed for your base level of Maslow's Hierarchy of survival. Your inner (or actual) husband looks out for where this money is sourced and strategizes, secures, and problem-solves so that you operate from a strong foundation.

So, if you're an entrepreneur or you long to be, hear me when I say, don't run naked into the fields too soon. Self-husband. Inspire your man to provide for you both. I believe that a man can only step into his true potential as a provider when a woman *stops contributing* and needs him to do just that. And if you don't have an able-bodied man, then use your imagination to secure a job that consistently pays the bills. Personally, when I was in $200k of debt after my medical training, I worked at the hospital for two years after I knew better. And then, when I decided that private practice wasn't for me any longer, I persisted until I knew my digital products were robust. These days, recurring revenue through memberships that I nurture represents my masculine money, there to pay my employees and keep the lights of my business on so my audacious whims are allowed to take flight. Give yourself a good foundation so that your creative magnetism can blossom and guide you on the spiral path of wealth.

247

Feminine money

This form of revenue could be defined by your ability to generate through your creative expression. This is the jewelry business you've been dreaming about starting, your somatic movement class you've been dying to offer, or your deep desire to grow and sell flowers by the bundle. It doesn't have to make sense; it just has to feel good, exciting, and magnetic to follow the path and ideas that would earn you feminine money. When you earn from this place, you are consistently doing so with sheer delight in the process, and you're creating for the sake of your God-given right to do so. When you are investing through a feminine lens, you are making a massive deposit into what I refer to as your vitality bank account; the ROI comes back in the form of the connection and expansion you *feel*.

I love thinking of money as a feminine energy that wants to come home and be well-cared for.

Here's the hard truth; You can really only be sustained entrepreneurially if you're tapped into your eros. The key to aligned success is in coming home to your body so you can use it as a navigational, intuitive instrument, rather than trying to force yourself to work in a way that doesn't work for you. With your eros reclaimed, you have the power to amplify your personal expression in the world. It feels completely different to make decisions entrepreneurially from a self-sourced, self-inspired space of trust than from scarcity, competition, and virtue-signaling.

In my own journey, I've witnessed the immense transformation available when you can expand the permission field, saying what would otherwise be considered completely audacious and wildly-off-the charts taboo, especially when it comes to doing business and making money. When you can smoke out the shadows of what keeps you trapped in kinky dynamics with money and creativity, the entrepreneurial possibilities are endless!

THE FIVE PERMISSION SLIPS OF AUDACIOUS ENTREPRENEURSHIP

Permission Slip 1: Own Your Stuckness

Before you can even begin to formulate a foundation for your definition of success, you must first legitimize the reason for your perceived stuckness. That means it's necessary for you to identify the chief complaint that you have, and then consider that there's a damn good reason that things are exactly the way you think you don't want them to be. Maybe you're a struggling single mom that feels trapped by your nine-to-five, or maybe you feel like you're constantly juggling too many balls as a one woman show, or maybe you just can't seem to book clients as a therapist, or you hire the world's most underqualified assistant, every time.

Take a moment to pause here and ask yourself:
What is my chief complaint right now?

From there, identify what it is that you "get to say" as a result of this chief complaint?
"Everybody else gets to have what they want but me."
"I never get to feel what it's like for someone to have my back"
"I have to do everything alone so it's harder for me"

Consider that there is a part of you inside that *needs* this problem in order to feel seen. When you can see and listen to this part and her victim story, the need to play it out diminishes, and new horizons become available. Remember that there is always a good reason that things are the way they are for you ... even if you think that you don't like it.

Permission Slip 2: Own Your Importance
Imposter syndrome plagues every expert, novice, and traveler on the road of self-expression. For many people in business, it's not easy to recognize their innate uniqueness because they imagine it's the content that matters, rather than the energy of its creation and delivery. That's why it can feel so empowering to understand why it has to be *you* that is offering what you're selling: you as the totality of all of your challenges, insights, growth, and

experience. Imposter syndrome resolves when you grow a strong spine and trust the solution that is channeled through your vessel. Whatever you do, just know that what you have to offer is important, and if you believe that, so will everyone else.

Permission Slip 3: Love Your Money
Because of our enculturation, it can feel too risky to admit that there is undoubtedly a part of you that wants money for the sake of money. The virtuous parts that say *I will do good with the money I get, I promise* and *I only want the money I need* often take the mic, but another quietly whispers *but it sure would be nice to have lots of it just to have it*. This permission slip is all about owning the part of you that actually *loves* wealth and the pleasure that comes with it. The part that translates wanting to having, whether it's a dress or a singing lesson or a dinner with friends. Get to know that part of you. Love that part of you and give her permission to play.

It's also helpful to know how you will receive the money and feel its fullness and its *telos*. What do you get when you have it? And what do you get because of having that? How will it make you feel? And how will you know when you've actually met that marker of success within yourself? Will it be because of the number in your bank account? Will it be because you can buy yourself fresh roses by the dozen every day of the week? Or finally afford to fly all your besties to the Outlander tour in Scotland? Get curious around the apologetic desire for money and how, in the light of day, that desire transforms into true creative potential.

Permission Slip 4: Barely Work
There is a pre-programmed shame-based belief that says, "If you work really hard, then you get to have it. If you don't, then you don't, because other people are." This is such a deep program, one that you might not even

know is operating until you start to dive into this work. It's also one that's so imperative to debunk so you can land in the deliciousness of *softpreneurship.*

What if you decide that you want your monthly bare minimum revenue to be $50,000, and you are only working two hours a week for that? It's probable that alarm bells sound off inside you that shout, *oh no, that's not possible, and I couldn't handle what people will say about me?!* This is why I often say, "Your haters are your gurus." The negative commentary you might receive around your capacity to earn effortlessly will showcase what you so deeply need to reclaim within yourself.

Notice the reflexive part of you that feels pressured to "explain" and legitimize your work through how "hard" you worked to receive the reward. Work smarter, not harder, woman! And own that you're smart enough to earn your own leisure. The next time someone makes a snide comment dressed as a compliment, recognize it as their desire and observe your ability to sit with it. Notice what comes up and see if you can simply say "thank you."

Permission Slip 5: Be a bad wrong, broke failure that no one likes (a.k.a. love your parts)

Let's revisit all the beautiful work you've done around wearing your inner Villain Crown. This permission slip is about getting comfortable with people thinking, saying, and feeling all kinds of potentially displeasing things about you. Become comfortable with doing it wrong, fucking it up, even embarrassing yourself in public. You *could* accidentally say something the wrong way, or otherwise be a failure that nobody likes. Big whoop! Because as you know by now, there are parts of you that are protecting you from social abandonment, rejection, and betrayal, but now, *you've got you,* and those parts can be reassigned to new duties.

If there are parts of you that *already* believe these things, you can shortcut your process, drain the drama, and alchemize the shame into lightness and humor. Can you let that narrative live? Can you own the part of you that agrees with your worst critic? Consciously and intentionally visiting with the absolute most feared condemnation can liberate you from the vigilant brace against it. Try it on, consider it, and see what happens if you let it be true, inside yourself, for just a few moments. You might find that the part of you holding that belief exhales some eros back into your system.

CHAPTER 15

Women's Hands

The time with Wild Woman is hard at first . . . [It] takes a boundless and mystical endurance. When we come up out of the underworld after one of our undertakings there, we may appear unchanged outwardly, but inwardly we have reclaimed a vast and womanly wildness. On the surface we are still friendly but beneath the skin, we are most definitely no longer tame.

—Dr. Clarissa Pinkola Estés[1]

Regeneration

As the maiden was welcomed in by the women of the cottage, the young king returned to his castle across the land. Even if his child was half-dog, the king could find no place in his heart to reject his son. Full of joyful anticipation to see his wife and the child, he was stunned to hear that they were dead. His mother showed him the deer eyes and tongues that she had been told her son demanded, only to be shocked by his spontaneous expression of grief. His wise mother realized that the devil must have mixed the messages, so she showed him the message that had supposedly come from him, telling her to kill his bride and newborn child and cut out their eyes and tongues. Reinvigorated, he sprang into action to find them, and still clothed in his battle garb, he set out again, determined never to rest until they were reunited. In her wisdom, the king's mother watched him go with pride, knowing it was her son's time to face the forest and become acquainted with its mysterious alchemical ways.

The king searched high and low, trodding through the woods carefully, sharing space with the shadowy wolves and giving a wide berth to foraging bears. His beard grew long and full as the rest of him withered down to nerve and sinew, caked in mud. Wild as the beasts who roamed alongside him, he searched for his lost wife and child for nearly seven years.

Amazingly, steeped in the beautiful community of woods women in the cottage, the maiden's hands began to grow back. Regeneration was gradual at first; her hands growing slowly as she sang in a circle of women, or a sister braided her hair, or when she danced in the meadow with dew on her dress at sunrise. Her fingers got longer as she nursed her son, bathed him in streams, and even raised those tender growing hands to protect him from a bear. At first, she had the hands of a baby, soft, sweet, and fumbling. Then she watched them grow into the hands of a child as she learned to cook, to knit, to dig in the earth. Within months, adolescent hands that were more dexterous mastered the harp, and she learned to sing new songs. Eventually, where her stumps had been, she saw her womanly hands again, only now she knew how important they were. The maiden and her hands fully regenerated in the community of woods women, all while her king searched on.

One fateful twilight, the king saw smoke and heard the low bawdy laughter of young men. Out hunting, the men were drinking ale and enjoying a heavenly spring evening, when the earth was ripe with possibility. They welcomed the wild king, feeding him and refilling his mug of ale. In their presence, he felt revived, once more a part of the brotherhood, surrounded by raucous tales and ribald jokes, invigorated by their masculine presence. He soon began to feel hopeful, and for the first time in years, his voice came out, dry and hoarse from disuse. "I'm looking for a woman without hands. And a young boy."

The men knew who she was, for the women of the woods were their family and their loves. With a lighter heart and comforted mind, the wild king washed off the surface layer of forest in a nearby stream, preparing to reunite with his love.

The men and women's lodges arranged a reunion. For a brief moment, a veil was raised between husband and wife, and when it was lowered, they peered into one another's souls. Looking with pure curiosity, wonder and love, they saw what seven years in the forest had given them: a deep initiation into the landscape of their wild, individuated Selves, like gems polished through endurance, challenge, grace, and a dash of magic. Though the king thought his heart couldn't be any fuller, it almost burst with love and joy as he saw his young son, standing by his mother's side, clutching one of her newly regrown hands. He took her other hand, reviewing the new skin with amazed reverence. He was complete.

Never before had anyone witnessed a night of such merriment and revelry, and never since, as intoxicating love poured forth as they renewed their vows: with each other and within themselves. The *heiros gamos*, marriage of the torn-asunder psychic polarities, complete.

Reclaiming Your Hands

The beauty of this tale is astounding; the maiden grows her hands back in the community of women. Doesn't it stir a truth deep within your soul?

When the maiden finds the cottage of women, she beholds their wisdom, their connection with the forest and each other, and the strength and protection symbolized by the men who love them, and finally understands what all the heartache and struggle was for. The loss of her hands has forced her to grow into more than just her father's daughter; finding and losing her king has proven that she was always strong enough to hold herself, and now she can choose to truly receive. She comes to see exactly why she said *Yes* to her self-initiation replete with rupture, hardship, and shadow-hunting through the *No*, discovering new levels of expansion again and again. And just as her inner feminine has been forged through trials, her inner king must mature through a masculine initiation of hardship, wearing his grief in his beard, weathering his hands and sharpening his instincts, until he is rewarded in sacred masculine community, man enough now for his forest queen.

They grow together, yet separately, into wholeness.

It is with other women that we are meant to walk that solo journey home to Self. As a woman, I can walk in the dark, and in the moments that I reach my hands forward, I feel hers and hers and hers there to gently guide me. I can thank my second marriage for inspiring me to button up my sexual energy and turn toward sisterhood, and I can thank those women for offering me the containment needed to walk through the hardest loss of my life when the fantasy of that marriage was exposed. It was women in my life, and it *is* women in my life, who support my permission field of becoming. I've needed other women, all kinds of women, to give me permission to try on new habits, types of behavior, and ways of being, to alchemize shame, and to inspire me toward my deepest initiations to date:

- To have more hard real talks with my family of origin
- To let go of the things I thought I'd die without
- To soften my hardest activist edicts
- To let my daughters be their own women
- To free my voice and dance in new ways
- To say "No" when I felt a little *no* and "Yes" when I felt a little *yes*

What I've learned from expressing feelings through my body is that I am here, dancing with myself, sharing with you what that's like, and longing to know what it's like for you to dance with yourself, so that we can dance with ourselves, together.

When you are around women who have light and energy moving through their vessel, it invites your body to remember, and your eros is freed from vaults and catacombs of detention. There is no greater medicine than the remembrance of a woman showing up for herself in the loving presence of other women doing the same.

It's notable that when women come together, we often cry. I can barely recall an instance where I've gathered women around me—to talk business, enjoy a potluck, or dance together—where there haven't been tears. It's not an accident that crying is a diagnostic criterion for Major Depressive Disorder, yet another vital experience of the human body pathologized and maligned. But as my ally, Veda Austin the water whisperer, says in our Reclamation Radio podcast interview: "Your tears trace a path from your eyes to your mouth because *they are your own medicine.*"

Your heart wants to feel safe to exist, to channel, and to express. And you can offer this safety to yourself while the women around you gaze upon you with knowing eyes that say, *you've got you.* In fact, I believe that's all I've ever done for women as a practitioner with remarkable outcomes; I've held steady the vision of a woman's grandeur even when she cannot see it. I've put a hand out in the dark, knowing she will find it.

There will come a time where we are called to consciousness and compelled to choose a deeper connection to ourselves over the false security of the poor bargain. Let's normalize this archetypal journey together, and let's model for our daughters what it looks like to become the woman that you were always meant to be.

In coming together in this movement, rising beyond our feminist programming, we liberate ourselves from disempowered, disconnected, resentful shells. We emerge, vital, pulsing vessels of sacred energy, with a strong, loving gaze trained on exactly that which we seek to alchemize into delight, abundance, and pleasure.

The approval that we offer one another as women models the authentic approval of the self, and this approval allows our shame-holding part to come out into the light and find a new job, perhaps, as the cheerleader holding enthusiasm for change. If up until now you've had trouble finding or connecting with the community of women who understand you, know that they are waiting for you, that your spirit in white will guide you to them just as it guided you here. And there is more where this came from . . .

This is a movement, and we are its co-creators. I'm growing my hands of self-nurturance and self-acceptance back, so that you can feel me reaching them out to you, woman.

VISUALIZATION: YOUR HOME IN COMMUNITY

Go ahead and clear your mind, preparing to visualize.

Imagine that you just woke up, but you have no clue where you are.

You do know that it's cold. In fact, there's snow all around, and you seem to be in a forest. And as if that weren't disorienting enough, it's also getting dark.

You stumble to your feet, feeling more scared and anxious by the minute, as your heart starts to race and you realize that you don't know what to do. You spot a path through the woods, carefully formed by a few unknown feet. Without any other obvious options, you choose the path as your next move and follow it as it winds through the darkening wood.

You don't know how long you follow this path, alternating between walking and jogging as you feel the dark press closer.

Just as it usually does in this kind of story, a clearing suddenly appears before you, and in it you see light coming through the windows of a house.

You almost collapse with relief. You're going to be okay.

As you get closer to the house, you see a man standing outside the door, and when he looks at you, it feels like he *knows* you. Not like a friendly face at church or in the grocery store, but like an old friend deeply invested in your wellbeing.

He smiles and invites you into the house.

Inside, the house is bursting with women and girls. And they're all sooo excited to see you.

One of them, a beaming sixteen-year-old, invites you to come sit with her, and guides you to a chair by the fire. She asks if she can braid your hair, and while her gentle fingers work the forest twigs and leaves from your hair, a motherly woman of forty brings you hot soup and bread, and it's the most delicious thing you've ever tasted, full of grandma's secrets and love, with just the right amount of salt.

You notice an older woman in the corner, but she's just observing all the bustle with a look of deeply contented satisfaction.

Before long, a little girl asks to sit on your lap, and she snuggles in, telling you a story she seems delighted by.

Looking around, it dawns on you why this house and its inhabitants feel so familiar.

All of these women and girls are *you*.

They're you at different stages of your life, from fresh-faced innocent to sage old wise woman, and all the incarnations in between.

And they fucking love you. They love you so much.

And they want your love and attention.

Suddenly it feels like there's nowhere else you'd rather be.

Now, come out of the visualization.

Feel that man outside. He's the strong container for you—the you that you *are*—made up of the sixteen-year-old maiden, the forty-year-old matron, the sweet-faced child, the happy, content granny, and more.

I want you to feel his energy up your spine, his knowing gaze, his righteous fucking boundaries and devotional attentiveness.

And I want you to feel all of that feminine energy swirling around inside, literally, and figuratively, as flavors of you-ness.

A woman alive, a Reclaimed Woman, is the most powerful force on this plane. Simply by choosing to feel, to honor her body, and to express her creativity, she inspires right action in herself and in those around her, and she breaks the spell of victimhood and the endless churn of struggle and suffering in the world. When her channels are open, she is running God through her body every day, all day, choosing life rather than bracing against pain and rejecting what is in front of her. She laughs, she screams, she cries, she kisses, she caresses. She is prismatic and kinetic. She both nurtures and destroys in the name of love.

So, let's remember what we came here for and why we incarnated into these beautiful bodies. Let's feel, sense, and breathe. Let's relate to all our own inner dimensions with curiosity and compassion. Let's end the war with men. Let's enjoy wealth, pleasure, and play. Let's finally be the mamas who know that love starts with self. Let's walk audaciously in the dark, on the edge of the wild unknown. Now is the time to end the cycles that your motherline handed down to you and to recognize the power of your intuition, your voice, and your sensuality to change the resonant frequency of every aspect of your life, from mothering to romance to business.

Welcome to your *Yes!* You have arrived.

In my group containers, I often offer a poem by "Wise at Heart" called *"Ou es tu?"* as in the French phrase, *where are you?* An extraordinarily beautiful and deeply touching work, it echoes the refrain of Maya Angelou's poem, "Still I rise." It opens my channel wide and reconnected, and I weep with the ineffability of what it is to be a woman in this life.

Create some space to truly receive the transmission of this powerful wordscape. Consider this a devotional offering from my heart to yours, inviting you to honor the full spectrum of your inner feminine, in all her many shades.

"OU ES TU?"
By Wise at Heart

Where are you, little girl with broken wings but full of hope? Where are you, wise woman covered in wounds?

Where are you? Where are you? Where are you?

Today is the day I will not sit still and give in anymore; today I rise.

I am bruised but I will get up and walk again; today I rise. I don't care if you ignore my beauty; today I rise.

Through the alchemy of my darkest night, I heal and thrive; today I rise.

I move through the world with confidence and grace. I open my eyes and am ready to face my wholeness as a woman and my limitless capacities. I will walk my path with audacity; today I rise.

I reconnect with the many aspects of myself. I am in awe of the reality I can create. I am a queen, I am a healer, a wise woman, a wild woman. I will rise and be.

I am a rebel. I will wake up and fight. I am a mother and I am a child. I will no longer disguise my sadness and pain; I will no longer suffer and complain. I am black and I am white. There's no reason to hide.

Where are you? Where are you?

I call upon Kali to kiss me to life. I transform my power and anger: no more heartache or strife. The world is missing what I am ready to give, my wisdom, my sweetness, my love, and my hunger for peace.

I weep with the trees and the rivers and the earth in distress. I rise and shine and am ready to go on my quest.

Today I rise without doubt or hesitation, today I rise without excuses, without procrastination.

Today I call upon my sisters to join a movement of resoluteness and concern. Today is my call into action, to fulfill your mission without further distraction.

Today is the day, today I will start to offer the world the wisdom of my heart.

261

"Thank You" is My Prayer

My best friend Tahra is my soul traveler, and we've journeyed together over a million rebirths since our rollerblade gang on Heights Road back when we were eleven years old. She's offered me a trove of gems, and one is that "'thank you' is a prayer." In fact, it is *how* to pray.

So, with that in mind, heart, and creative centers, I offer a closing prayer . . .

Thank you, body, for the way you respond to all that is asked of you.

Thank you to my thinking, toiling, and ever-vigilant mind and to all the clarity it yields.

Thank you to all the feelings I came here to feel and to the perfect-as-is stories that allow me to feel them.

Thank you to all my parts—the protectors, the child fragments, and the managers—for your most benevolent intentions.

Thank you to each and every persecutor, OP, and villain who gave my inner victim a juicy tale to tell, and feelings of fear, rage, and grief to feel into completion.

Thank you to conflict, adversity, disease, and all the horrors and hurts of humanity for helping to inspire a fierce yearning for remedy, regeneration, and remembrance.

Thank you to the children who are the spiritual leaders of the next chapter masquerading as helpless dependents.

Thank you to the animals who are angels guarding our hearts.

Thank you to each and every woman. The ones I've loved and the ones I've judged.

Thank you to the chain of mothers serving up the perfect ingredients for reclamation across generations.

Thank you to the men for your service, your courage, and your strength, and for making and building all the things you make and build.

Thank you to the women gathering with women and the men gathering with men.

Thank you to the beautiful, committed couples in sacred union guarding the man-woman dyad.

Thank you to anyone making anything with your hands, singing with your voice, dancing with your body.

Thank you to the wisdom keepers and deep thinkers.

Thank you to the early adopters and vanguard envelope pushers for giving me permission to risk approval for what feels true and real.

Thank you to each and every one of you for holding your creative spark, following your wild and weird impulses, and expressing your gifts even before they feel ripe and ready.

Thank you to every damn person owning their shit and their grandeur.

Thank you to you, dear woman, for walking this audacious path home, with me.

Acknowledgments

And while I'm expressing my gratitude . . . Thank you:

To the manuscript midwives! Elyssa Jakim for the delightful process of weaving this work into being, Alyssa Jarvi for your erudite review and for the "Handless Maiden" inspo, Dawn Petrin and Meli Neubek for your loving oversight.

Whitney Lowery for midwifing *me* into my pleasure and beyond the pain of my victim tales.

Leela Lorenzoni for being the sister/cousin alongside and behind every iteration of me, my creations, and all that wants to become through our epic business.

Jamie Davidson for your soul partnership in the field of reclamation.

Meli Neubek, Lismany Medina, Talia Behrend, and Julie LoGreco as well as Scott McDermott, Suzanne Moscovitch, Elyssa Jakim and Dawn Petrin and AllConnected, Katie Hess, and Lotus Wei for your devoted support of all things KBMD.

Audacious Embodiment girlies including Simone Sobers, Wendy Diaz, Kimi Inch, Daniela Garcia, Akasha, Amerly, River Roaring, Ellie, Madelyn Moon, Hanna Leigh, and an honorary Dominique and Kukuwa for being the marriage officiants of my parts at the wedding party of my dreams!

Sarah Kamrath, Eyla Cuenca, Jamie Kozisek-Johnson, Akasha, Atalya Starre, Claudia Morales, Whitney Burrell, Daniela Garcia, Isa Herrera, Maya Shetreat, and Patricia Hart for holding my feminine essence with grace, beauty, and play.

Sofia Fink for the exquisite delight that it is to be in your presence, to expand through your preternatural wisdom, to laugh with you, explore with you, and be weird together.

Lucia Fink for your sacred innocence, loveliness, your affection, your dance moves, and for the emotional sophistication, soulfulness, and self-allegiance that you have exemplified since your birth.

Noah Dresden, Natalia, and Bryan for bringing beautiful love into my Sofia's life.

Tahra Collins for pinning the fabric of my reality in love, over all of these decades.

Amerly Centeno for your huge heart and endless wisdom in constellating my Self, family, and loved ones.

Andy Fink for being the baby-daddy I choose in this life and to Lauren for supporting him.

Marusca Brogan for your huge heart, playfulness, wisdom, and Italian fire.

VLP and VMR warriors for standing with me, for Your Self.

Ron Brogan for all the ways that I needed to anchor masculine virtues including integrity of word, follow through, wise action, loyalty, and presence.

Bren Brogan for your kindness, forgiveness, and steady presence.

Nick Gonzalez, Nonnie, and Sharkey for your etheric presence in my lifescape.

Tom Cowan for being exactly the man I needed to show up at exactly the time you did so that I could remember how to love myself through the eyes of a trusted father figure, for your incisive mind, and for your incessant jokes.

Om Rupani, Tom Holmes, and Kirby Hotchner for your specific masculine support in critical windows of my journey.

Joseph for being my house-husband handyman extraordinaire!

Sayer for showing up with the exact alchemical ingredients needed to catalyze my journey home to love.

The Friday Group for offering me a sense of true belonging (and sanity). You know who you are: $8''/mi^2$

Mushi, Bitty, the chickens, and Puffykitty for giving my inner girl all she's ever wanted.

Skyhorse for taking me in when no other publisher would.

Becca of Skye High Designs for the most beautiful book cover ever!

To all the long-timers who have stood by cheering on my breakdown breakthroughs and loving me even as I've evolved, I deeply thank you for your gaze . . .

Endnotes

Introduction
1 Jason D. Wright, et al. "Scientific evidence underlying the American College of Obstetricians and Gynecologists' practice bulletins." *Obstetrics and gynecology* vol. 118,3 (2011): 505-512. doi:10.1097/AOG.0b013e3182267f43.
2 "Outcomes." n.d., https://www.kellybroganmd.com/outcomes.

Chapter 1
1 Clarissa Pinkola Estés, *Women Who Run with the Wolves: Myths and Stories of the Wild Woman Archetype* (New York: Ballantine Books,1992).
2 Ibid, 426–427.
3 Alexander Lowen, *Fear of Life* (Hinesburg, VT: The Alexander Lowen Foundation, 2012).

Chapter 2
1 Daniel Estulin, *Tavistock Institute: Social Engineering the Masses* (Walterville, OR: Trine Day, 2015).
2 Sigmund Freud, *Mass Psychology (Penguin Modern Classics Translated Texts).* (Penguin UK, 2004).
3 Louise Perry, *The Case Against the Sexual Revolution* (Polity Press, 2022).
4 Ibid, 9.
5 Ibid, 14.
6 I have followed David Deida's teachings for years and you'll notice his work in the polarity space informs this book and have mostly studied his lectures. For David Deida's core teachings, you can explore his many books and recordings. My recommended starting place is the book *Intimate Communion*.
7 David Deida "The Official David Deida Website." n.d., accessed August 11, 2022. https://deida.info/.
8 Lowen, *Fear of Life.*

Chapter 3
1 Lindsay C. Gibson, *Adult Children of Emotionally Immature Parents* (New Harbinger Publications, 2016).
2 Alfie Kohn, *Unconditional Parenting: Moving from Rewards and Punishments to Love and Reason* (New York: Atria Books, 2006).

3   Gibson, *Adult Children of Emotionally Immature Parents.*
4   Ibid, 27.
5   Ibid, 70.
6   Ibid, 28.
7   Bruce K. Alexander, et al. "Effect of Early and Later Colony Housing on Oral Ingestion of Morphine in Rats." *Pharmacology Biochemistry and Behavior* 15 (4): 571–76 (1981). https://doi.org/10.1016/0091-3057(81)90211-2.
8   Jean Liedloff, *The Continuum Concept* (London: Penguin, 2009).
9   Sam Vaknin, "Narcissist-Abuse," Narcissistic-Abuse.com., n.d., accessed April 11, 2024. https://www.narcissistic-abuse.com/.

Chapter 4
1   Friedrich Wilhelm Nietzsche, Helen Zimmern, and Robert Silverrider, *Beyond Good and Evil: Prelude to a Philosophy of the Future,* 1886.
2   Steven A. Young, *A Fool's Wisdom: Science Conspiracies & the Secret Art of Alchemy.* Independently Published, 2024.
3   Thomas Cowan, Letter to Kelly Brogan. Email, 2022.
4   Stephen Karpman, "The Official Site of the Karpman Drama Triangle," 2014. https://karpmandramatriangle.com/.

Chapter 5
1   Carolyn Elliott, *Existential Kink: Unmask Your Shadow and Embrace Your Power* (Newburyport, MA: Weiser Books, 2020).
2   Ibid, 102.
3   Jack Morin, *The Erotic Mind* (Harper Perrenial, 1995).
4   Elliott, *Existential Kink: Unmask Your Shadow and Embrace Your Power.*

Chapter 6
1   CG Jung and RFC Hull, *Dreams* (London: Routledge Classics, 2002).
2   Lynne Forrest and Eileen Meagher, *Guiding Principles for Life beyond Victim Consciousness* (Chattanooga, TN: Conscious Living Media, 2011).

Chapter 7
1   Pinkola Estés, *Women Who Run with the Wolves: Myths and Stories of the Wild Woman Archetype.*
2   Ibid, 451.
3   Ibid, 460.
4   Marion Woodman, *Conscious Femininity* (Inner City Books, 1993).
5   Pinkola Estés, *Women Who Run with the Wolves: Myths and Stories of the Wild Woman Archetype.*
6   Taisha Abelar, *The Sorcerer's Crossing* (Penguin, 1993).
7   Robert Gilbert, *Spiritual Science: Essential Teachings & Practices* (2013).
8   John Kreiter, *Vampire's Way to Psychic Self-Defense* (Createspace Independent Publishing Platform, 2016).

Chapter 8

1 Whitney Lowery, "Somatic Experiencing Practices." n.d.

Chapter 9

1 Richard C. Schwartz, *No Bad Parts: Healing Trauma and Restoring Wholeness with the Internal Family Systems Model* (Boulder, Colorado: Sounds True, 2021).
2 Ibid, 25.
3 Ibid, 26.
4 Amerly Centeno, "Quanta Academy." Quanta Academy LLC., n.d., accessed April 11, 2024. https://quantasystemicacademy.com/.

Chapter 10

1 Daniela Garcia, "The Joy Alchemist," The Joy Alchemist, n.d., accessed April 11, 2024. https://www.the-joy-alchemist.com/.
2 Peter A. Levine, *Somatic Experiencing : Esperienze Somatiche Nella Risoluzione Del Trauma* (Roma: Astrolabio Ubaldini, 2014).
3 Kimi Inch, "Erotic Leadership," Reclamation Radio, 2024.
4 Om Rupani, *Prerequisites to Ecstasy* (2017).
5 Andreas A.J. Wismeijer and Marcel A.L.M. van Assen, "Psychological Characteristics of BDSM Practitioners," *The Journal of Sexual Medicine* 10 (8) (2013): 1943–52. https://doi.org/10.1111/jsm.12192.
6 Elise Wuyts and Manuel Morrens, "The Biology of BDSM: A Systematic Review," *The Journal of Sexual Medicine* 19 (1)(2022): 144–57. https://doi .org/10.1016/j.jsxm.2021.11.002.
7 Elise Wuyts, et al., "Between Pleasure and Pain: A Pilot Study on the Biological Mechanisms Associated with BDSM Interactions in Dominants and Submissives," *The Journal of Sexual Medicine* 17 (4)(2020): 784–92. https://doi.org/10.1016/j.jsxm.2020.01.001.
8 Stephanie Pappas, "The New Yoga? Sadomasochism Leads to Altered States, Study Finds." Livescience.com., February 19, 2014, https://www.livescience .com/43502-sadomasochism-mind-alteration.html.
9 Lizette Borreli, "S&M May Be the New Yoga: BDSM Causes Blood Flow in Brain to Alter State of Consciousness," *Medical Daily*, February 21, 2014, https://www.medicaldaily.com/sm-may-be-new-yoga-bdsm-causes-blood -flow-brain-alter-state-consciousness-269863.
10 Charlotta Carlström, "BDSM, Becoming and the Flows of Desire," *Culture, Health & Sexuality* 21 (4)(2018): 404–15. https://doi.org/10.1080/13691058.2 018.1485969.
11 Brad J. Sagarin, et al., "Hormonal Changes and Couple Bonding in Consensual Sadomasochistic Activity," *Archives of Sexual Behavior* 38 (2) (2008): 186–200. https://doi.org/10.1007/s10508-008-9374-5.
12 Cory J. Cascalheira, et al., "Curative Kink: Survivors of Early Abuse Transform Trauma through BDSM," *Sexual and Relationship Therapy* 38 (3) (2021): 1–31. https://doi.org/10.1080/14681994.2021.1937599.

Chapter 11

1 Pinkola Estés, *Women Who Run with the Wolves: Myths and Stories of the Wild Woman Archetype*.

2 Martin Shaw, *Smoke Hole: Looking to the Wild in the Time of the Spyglass* (White River Junction, VT: Chelsea Green Publishing, 2021).

3 Pinkola Estés, *Women Who Run with the Wolves: Myths and Stories of the Wild Woman Archetype*.

4 Ibid, 482.

5 It's worth noting that regarding the communities of men and women featured in Martin Shaw's telling of the tale, Estés offers a different variation. The variation of the story with a veil being lifted between husband and wife also appears in Shaw's telling of the tale. Shaw, Smokehole, 49–50.

6 Pinkola Estés, *Women Who Run with the Wolves: Myths and Stories of the Wild Woman Archetype*.

Chapter 12

1 Mama Gena, "Home," Mama Gena, n.d., accessed April 11, 2024. https://mamagenas.com/.

2 Elliott, *Existential Kink: Unmask Your Shadow and Embrace Your Power*.

3 Whitney Lowery, "Somatic Experiencing Practices," n.d.

4 Kasia Urbaniak, "Welcome to the Academy: The School of Power for Women," n.d., accessed April 11, 2024. https://www.kasiaurbaniak.com/.

Chapter 13

1 Betty Martin and Robyn Dalzen, *The Art of Receiving and Giving: The Wheel of Consent* (Eugene, OR: Luminare Press, 2021).

2 Betty Martin, "The Wheel of Consent," YouTube, 2014. https://www.youtube.com/watch?v=auokDp_EA80.

3 Martin and Dalzen, *The Art of Receiving and Giving: The Wheel of Consent*.

4 Betty Martin, "How to Play the 3-Minute Game," YouTube, 2016. https://www.youtube.com/watch?v=_KCzpNBNbVM.

5 Betty Martin, "Betty Martin – Developer of the Wheel of Consent," Bettymartin.org., n.d., accessed April 11, 2024, https://bettymartin.org/.

6 Jaiya, "Erotic Blueprints and Breakthrough with Jaiya," Miss Jaiya.com, n.d., https://missjaiya.com/.

Chapter 14

1 Pia Mellody, Andrea Wells Miller, and Keith Miller, *Facing Love Addiction: Giving Yourself the Power to Change the Way You Love* (New York: HarperOne, Enfield, 2010).

2 David Deida, "The Official David Deida Website," n.d., accessed August 11, 2022. https://deida.info/.

3 Laura Doyle, *The Surrendered Wife: A Practical Guide for Finding Intimacy, Passion and Peace with a Man* (London: Pocket, 2006).

4   Susan M. Johnson, et al., "Soothing the Threatened Brain: Leveraging Contact Comfort with Emotionally Focused Therapy," edited by Kevin Paterson, *PLoS ONE* 8 (11)(2013.): e79314. https://doi.org/10.1371/journal.pone.0079314.

Chapter 15
1   Pinkola Estés, *Women Who Run with the Wolves: Myths and Stories of the Wild Woman Archetype*.

271

For reclamation-related freebies related to my masterclasses, podcast episodes, and my Audacious Activation Challenge, scan here:

Or visit
www.kellybroganmd.com/rwfreebies